M000211150

Mindful
Menopause

202066666

About the Author

For over 15 years Sophie has been a clinical hypnotherapist and Fellow of the National Council for Hypnotherapy. She specialises in our unconscious responses to change. Having written a thesis on psyche, symbolism and language for her Masters she went on to train in therapy focused on women's psychological well-being during the transitions of birth, motherhood and menopause. This is her third book and follows the bestselling *Mindful Hypnobirthing* and *Mindful Mamma*. She also contributed to the *Here and Now* audiobook. All her work is about creating simple, nurturing, practical tools for positive psychological change.

You can find and connect with Sophie online at www.mindfulmenopause.co.uk or on Instagram @mindful_menopause.

Mindful Menopause

How to have a calm and positive menopause

SOPHIE FLETCHER

Vermilion
LONDON

Vermilion, an imprint of Ebury Publishing,
20 Vauxhall Bridge Road,
London SW1V 2SA

Vermilion is part of the Penguin Random House group of companies
whose addresses can be found at global.penguinrandomhouse.com

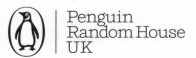

Penguin
Random House
UK

Copyright © Sophie Fletcher 2021

Illustrations © Michele Donnison 2021

Sophie Fletcher has asserted her right to be identified as the author of
this Work in accordance with the Copyright, Designs and Patents Act 1988

First published by Vermilion in 2021

www.penguin.co.uk

A CIP catalogue record for this book is available from the British Library

ISBN 9781785042942

Printed and bound in Great Britain by Clays Ltd, Elcograf S.p.A.

The authorised representative in the EEA is Penguin Random House
Ireland, Morrison Chambers, 32 Nassau Street, Dublin D02 YH68.

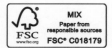

Penguin Random House is committed to
a sustainable future for our business, our readers
and our planet. This book is made from Forest
Stewardship Council® certified paper.

The information in this book has been compiled as general guidance on the specific subjects addressed. It is not a substitute and not to be relied on for medical, healthcare or pharmaceutical professional advice. Please consult your GP before changing, stopping or starting any medical treatment. So far as the author is aware the information given is correct and up to date as at March 2021. Practice, laws and regulations all change and the reader should obtain up-to-date professional advice on any such issues. The author and publishers disclaim, as far as the law allows, any liability arising directly or indirectly from the use or misuse of the information contained in this book.

For you, yes you!

This book is dedicated to everything that you have
done and everything you will continue to do that makes
you the strong, wise and capable woman you are.

WEST SUSSEX LIBRARY SERVICE	
202066666	
Askews & Holts	23-Jul-2021
612.665	

I do not wish women to have power over men;
but over themselves.

Mary Wollstonecraft

Contents

CONTENTS

Introduction

Teach us to care and not to care.

T.S. Eliot

This was a book I *had* to write. I've worked in women's health, particularly around transitions, for the last 15 years. As I started to go through menopause myself, I discovered first-hand just how powerful the tools I use are for this life stage.

Many of the women I see in my practice are post-menopausal, or in the late stages of perimenopause (the transition stage leading up to menopause), but this isn't why they come to me. They often come for help with issues such as lack of sleep, weight gain and sudden onset anxiety. I quickly made the connection between the experiences that those women were having and their life stage. In working with them, I learned how individual each experience is.

I know from my own experience that preparation and knowledge are key to a good menopause. It's much easier to make those adjustments and changes when you know what is happening to your body and what you can do to support those changes in a positive way.

That's not to say that there is a magic wand. I know how hard perimenopause can hit – my hair fell out in handfuls, and at one point I had a monk's crown! But people comment on my positive attitude, and it's true that mindset makes all the difference. The impact of unconscious thoughts and feelings cannot be underestimated and how I thought about it helped me to respond to it.

In my early 40s, I knew that preparing by adapting and making lifestyle changes would benefit me in the long run. Some of these were simple self-care changes, but others were harder, like changing lifelong attitudes to diet and exercise. I also become disciplined in my meditation practice, something that had been harder as a new parent, but which was easier as my children grew into adults.

We tend to think of menopause as a very physical experience, and a lot of the time it is, but it's so much more. It's a transition from one life stage to another. Like all transitions, it can be powerful and exhilarating, but also tough. There will be days when you just about stay afloat, knowing that day will pass. Experiences can be physical, emotional or spiritual – and sometimes, all of those things, at the same time! No wonder it's a roller-coaster.

A note about terminology

Did you know that menopause, as medically defined, is just one day of your life? It's officially the 365th day after your last period. Often you might hear people say, 'I'm going through the menopause' and in truth if you have still had a period in the last 12 months, you are perimenopausal, which means 'around menopause'.

Culturally we talk about perinatal mental well-being, so for the sake of clarity and continuity I will refer to perimenopausal well-being, menopausal transition, or the time around menopause. This book is about your well-being around menopause, whether that spans years or months up to that 365th day after your last period.

Owning your experience

A menopausal transition isn't just a set of symptoms. In fact, in this book I don't use the word symptom. Instead, I refer to 'experiences' or 'expressions of menopause'. By doing this I'm inviting you to reassess your menopausal transition as something that you have control over, experience by experience. It is all new – each day that passes your hormones adjust and shift in different ways. Being tuned into this as a set of experiences creates a deeper connection with this transition to a new chapter. This is all about change – changes to your body, your life and your mindset.

A lot of menopause books discuss hormonal changes, what medication to take, what food to eat and the type of exercise that will benefit you. It's wonderful that this information is out there and gaining traction as it is needed, but the big question for me has always been 'How?' How do you make all those changes, when it sometimes means changing lifelong habits? How do you take all that information and make it part of your daily life without it feeling overwhelming? In this book I'm going to show you the 'how'.

You may know what you should eat and what exercise you need to do; you may understand the importance of reducing stress. But if, like me, you have a busy life, finding the time to do this, and to get your head into a place where it's second nature, can be challenging.

This is the book that I was looking for and wanted to refer clients to, but that didn't exist until now. I've been encouraged to write it by my friends and clients who tell me 'everyone needs to know this!' Everything that I've learned from my own experiences and from working with my clients has been packed into these pages – creating a set of tailor-made practical tools to help you navigate these years, with confidence and calm.

Invaluable tools

There is so much that can be done with these tools and this type of approach. You're going to learn about mind–body connections, the unconscious triggers for certain aspects of menopause that can challenge you, and you're going to discover some great practical techniques to tackle underlying mental blocks around lifestyle changes such as diet and exercise. You'll also get practical mindset tools to help with feeling rested and energised, through to learning how you can manage anxiety and reduce hot flushes.

A calm and confident perimenopause is about creating good habits and daily rituals to support every aspect of your transition. In this book, I'll show you how to create them step by step in the easiest way possible.

Small adjustments create big changes, so if all you can do one day is stop and take a mindful breath, then that's great; you are noticing your need to stop and care for yourself. That in itself is a big deal! Other days you may want to get started on a journal, or a new routine – it's up to you. This is a great time to explore your creativity and this book can be a springboard for that.

Change starts earlier than you may think. Society needs to be having a conversation about preparation. We don't always see that change is happening until we are in the thick of it and need to do something – fast. Those early signs of perimenopause may be a snappy day with the children, feeling irritable or having a heavier than normal period. It may be the struggle and frustration of not being able to snap back to the size you are used to being. The shift can be sudden or gradual.

You can start to think practically about how you want to approach it, adapting it as necessary as you move forward. Like all transitions, this is a time of change, and where there is change growth happens. You have choices and can create your own narrative.

A time of possibility

'I feel liberated' is something that I hear time and time again. We don't always think of menopause as a time of possibility, but it is. It's also a time of creation, connection and collaboration. You are powerful, and you have everything you need within you to unfold gently and confidently into the next stage of your life.

My wish is that you take what you need from this book and make your menopause your own. If you just dip in and out and take a few nuggets that make you feel positive and inspired, perfect! If you read it cover to cover and feel a shift happening within you, then great! I'm not going to tell you what to do; I'm going to give you the tools to do what you feel is right for you.

I'm so glad that you are reading these words and you have this book in your hands. You now have the opportunity to change your experience of perimenopause and what lies beyond. The journey you are about to embark on will create transformation where there is change and challenge. This book will help you ground yourself in the experience when you need to, grow from it when you are able and rest in it when you can. Most of all it's a celebration of who you are becoming and what you are capable of.

Sophie

How to Use This Book

This book is designed to be used from the early years of perimenopause right through to the day of your menopause and beyond. You can read it cover to cover, or you can dip in and out of the chapters that you feel drawn to, at any given moment. Make the book your own. Doodle in it, make notes, highlight your favourite phrases and exercises so you can come back to them easily.

There are affirmations scattered throughout the book and moments where you can just stop and have a mindful moment, to connect with your breath and a particular aspect of the book. I call these Meno-Pauses and I will prompt you to take them throughout with this symbol: ⑪. As you go through you may find that you make your own natural pauses, moments when you want to stop and reflect on a feeling or response to the words you have read.

You will need:

- A pen and notebook or journal to write notes and reflections.
- A device where you can download the audio tracks.
- Sticky notes for some of the exercises in the book.

The book is broken down into three parts:

Part 1: Your Menopause Toolkit

In this section you'll be introduced to the main tools that under-pin most of the exercises in the book. These will help you to become familiar with the aspects of mindfulness, meditation and hypnosis, which are perfect for perimenopause and beyond.

You'll learn about your calm menopause, how to do self-hypnosis visualisation and the value of a menopause journal.

Part 2: What's Going On? Mapping Your Menopause

Here you will learn about the aspects of menopause that are impacted by your thoughts and feelings. We'll take a brief look at your hormones, then explore aspects of your mind and body that can exacerbate your physical experiences of perimenopause and beyond. We'll delve into your thoughts and feelings, reflect on what this journey means, how you wish to experience it and how to get the support you need, whether at home or at work. Then you'll create a positive plan and intention for how you wish to experience your menopause and what that means to you.

Part 3: What You Can Do About It

This section tackles areas of menopause that I see most in my practice. With exercises, visualisations and tools that help you cool a hot flush, reduce anxiety, have a restful night or embrace your menopause body, you'll start to feel comfortable with using the techniques in the moments you need to. You can dip into these chapters as and when you need them. Finally, you have a Mindful Menopause checklist to help you integrate these tools into your daily life.

Online supporting material

There are a number of free audio tracks to download at www.penguin.co.uk/mindfulmenopause. These are explained in more depth as you go through the book. Look for the symbol. Please do not listen to these while driving.

- Your Calm Breath 45
- Grounding Yourself 58
- Starting Your Day With Joy 92
- Letting Go of Stress 122
- Growth Affirmations 132
- Reclaiming Your Power 144
- Hypnosis for Restorative Sleep 219
- Yoga Nidra 221
- Turning Down the Heat 231
- Intuitive Eating 286

This book is an invitation. Take what you want from it. There are over 75 exercises, but you don't have to do them all. Notice how you feel about them, which ones feel more intuitive and work well for you. They are all slightly different, but can be adapted. If there is one tool you love that is in a section that you may not need much help with, adapt it for something that you do need help with. The power of these tools is that you can make them your own.

Some of them may feel similar, but there are subtle differences between them and they are specific to certain aspects of midlife and menopause. Use the exercise list that follows to note which ones you found most useful and return to them.

List of exercises

Your Menopause Toolkit

1

What is a Mindful Menopause?

*I am the rest between two notes, which are
somehow always in discord.*

Rainer Maria Rilke

Rather than dreading this time of your life, imagine what it would be like to feel excited about the opportunities it gives you, and to know that you can tackle anything that arises anxiety-free. A mindful menopause will help you to do just that. It is a unique approach to perimenopause using a simple but effective blend of hypnosis and mindfulness tools, which will help you navigate this transition and respond to the challenges, whether physical, emotional or spiritual, in a positive way.

Never underestimate the power of the unconscious and your thoughts. A mindful menopause will show you the power of this mind–body connection and how you can use it in a way that lifts you up and makes you feel capable of achieving anything, while also helping to reduce your hot flushes!

Whether you are going through menopause with the help of Hormone Replacement Therapy (HRT) or are approaching it naturally, the changes that occur will affect you. Just as you were able to move through other life transitions and challenges, you will be able to move through this one, with more knowledge and experience than ever before.

This new transition is inevitable. And it can be exciting. The spiritual and emotional growth that is available to you right now may have been overshadowed by the patriarchal cultural narrative, not just of womanhood, but of menopause itself. So, let's start with a simple exercise to look at the story that plays in your mind around menopause.

EXERCISE 1: KNOWING YOUR NARRATIVE

Grab a pen and paper or use your journal. When you hear the word menopause, what three things come into your mind straight away? Allow your answers to be as spontaneous as possible. If you really have to think about answers 2 or 3, put your pen down and come back to the exercise later.

1. _____

2. _____

3. _____

We are going to look at this again at the end of the book.

The stories of what a 'menopausal woman is' that you have been told or that you tell yourself do not define who you are. *You* define who you are. You can choose to lean into this life transition and embrace the changes, learning to manage daily challenges with calm acceptance.

Imagine how wonderful it would be if you were able to let go of any doubts or expectations set in the past and embrace who you are right now, in this moment – a strong, wise, experienced woman. When you see all parts of yourself with kindness – and with honesty, forgiveness and love – you will connect deeply and authentically to your life and cultivate a warmth and wisdom, helping you to shine more brightly than you ever thought possible. I am going to help you towards this.

A multidimensional experience

The experience of menopause is multidimensional, not just physical. It can trigger bigger existential questions about life, such as 'Who am I?', 'How did I end up here?', 'What if I'd made that choice instead?' Some doors may feel closed, while others may be opening up.

Recognising and acknowledging these aspects of self will help you to become a friend to every part of you. And as you work through this book you may suddenly realise that you are beginning to lovingly embrace all aspects of who you are. It may be a 'wow' moment, or one day you may suddenly realise how much lighter and calmer you are feeling.

Accepting the parts of you that are anxious and fearful, as well as the parts that are warm and loving, will bring balance to your life and a level of contentment you may not have experienced before. This is a gift of menopause. It can be a time for healing and acceptance, and for making peace with who you are without having to 'be' someone for anyone else. Sometimes this can be difficult, sometimes easy; but growth doesn't happen without a challenge and in this moment, right now, you can allow yourself to embark on this journey to connect and know yourself in ways you may not have done before.

To do this, the techniques you are going to be getting to grips with are hypnosis, meditation and mindfulness. Let's dive in and get to know them.

All about hypnosis

When people discover I'm a hypnotherapist they often say, half-joking, 'I'm not going to look you in the eye!' The image they have in mind is the one they've seen on TV of spiralling eyes, swinging watches and a hypnotist controlling a person's every move. This is very far from the truth. As a hypnotherapist, I can't make you do anything you don't want to do – you are always in control of your own experience. My job is to guide you to achieve what you want in life. The tools I use help to bypass your inner procrastinator, critic and doubter.

Hypnosis isn't about being suggestible, but rather being open to suggestion, and open to the possibility of change. Suggestion is powerful. The easiest way to think of it is in the context of the placebo effect, which is when a dummy medicine has very similar effects to the real drug, sometimes even when the person knows it is fake. Whether you have back pain or a broken heart, thoughts and expectation can change your experience.

The work I do is always goal-driven and this is very important. It really focuses your mind on what matters to you and puts you in control. Whether it's changing a behaviour, habit or experience, you can explore ways of making that happen.

Hypnosis works best when people are open to the experience and engage with it wholeheartedly; when you trust that your mind is powerful enough to make changes you previously didn't think were possible. In the book you're going to learn how powerful belief and expectation can be, particularly when it comes to menopause.

You don't have to go to a hypnotherapist to benefit from hypnosis either. You can quickly learn self-hypnosis using the tools in this book.

What does it feel like?

Hypnosis is really relaxing. Most people are very surprised to find that it feels a little like having a comforting nap and describe it as a mind massage.

There are two types of hypnosis: state and non-state. State is the more formal type, when a hypnotherapist helps to guide you into a 'state of hypnosis'. I prefer to call it hypnotic relaxation. The tracks that accompany the book, such as the longer sleep tracks, are a form of state hypnosis.

Non-state is less formal. We are open to suggestion all of the time as we go about our daily lives. For example, I have interwoven this book with language for change. As you read it, you will feel calmer and more confident without really being able to put your finger on why. There are suggestions embedded in the text, some of which you won't take on board because they won't fit with your ideology, but others that align with your intention for a positive menopause.

With all kinds of hypnosis, there is evidence to show that expectation can affect the experience and success of hypnosis. This means that the more you believe that it will work, the more likely change will happen.

Hypnosis for menopause

Not many clients come to me for menopause hypnosis, well not intentionally! When I first started working as a hypnotherapist, I realised that many women, usually aged 45+, who came to my clinic had very similar complaints. Often things they had previously managed very easily suddenly seemed insurmountable – a common condition I saw was agoraphobia, fear of going out.

Feeling trapped was also a common experience that emerged. Sometimes it was just 'anxiety', but when we started to unpick it, there was often so much more beneath. Deeper philosophical questions would arise, childhood memories often resurfaced unexpectedly and generalised anxiety emerged. There was a deeper exploration of relationships, as these women adapted to life changes such as their children leaving home and faced fears about ageing and mortality for both themselves and their partner. Weight management was something else I found myself working with, particularly in women who have mobility problems relating to joint and bone changes.

It was very rare that women came to see me to help them around menopause. Why? Because people aren't aware that you can improve your experience of menopause with hypnotherapeutic techniques. In fact, I don't 'treat menopause' at all; instead, I work with individual issues that may arise for people at a particular life stage. Your experience will be different from every other woman – the most effective hypnosis should always be tailored to you, to *your* experience, beliefs and expectations.

There is good evidence of how hypnosis can support menopausal issues. One study showed that hot flushes can be reduced with simple visualisations, and there are numerous studies showing the effectiveness of hypnotherapy for weight management, anxiety, self-confidence, sexual confidence and enjoyment, and insomnia. There is even a small study that suggests improvements in hair growth.

Learning self-hypnosis will give you the resources to tailor and use the techniques on an ongoing basis. Understanding the theory and the research adds another dimension and can create a light-bulb moment. The power in learning how it works is in making it work for you.

The exercises and visualisations that you will learn in this book are superb tools that once understood can be applied effectively to a vast range of situations. All you need to do is be willing to jump in and give your imagination free reign. It will pay dividends.

Mindfulness and meditation

Many people are aware of the benefits of meditation and mindfulness to well-being. You may already have your own practice or have experienced it as part of a yoga class, or you may never have intentionally approached your life with mindfulness.

Mindfulness and meditation, although interwoven, are different. Meditation nurtures and helps embed your mindfulness practice. Mindfulness is like the rain that waters the meditation practice you cultivate.

Meditation is usually an intentional sitting practice. There are many different types of meditation, and they can last from five minutes to several hours. Some are calming and some are insightful. Some aim to embody wholehearted tenderness towards self and others, such as loving kindness, compassion or forgiveness. These can be known as 'Open Heart' meditations. Research shows that after eight weeks of regular meditation there are beneficial changes in your brain.

Mindfulness is a way to engage consciously with the world around you as you go about your daily life. Everything can be done with mindful awareness – for example, while you are washing the dishes, filling the car with fuel or drinking a cup of coffee, your mind is present, focused on the task or moment in hand. Mindfulness is loving, kind and free of judgement, and about being absolutely in the present. Try this simple mindfulness exercise . . .

EXERCISE 2: BEING PRESENT

Take a moment to be where you are right now. Notice your breathing – do not alter it in any way. Just notice. Now expand your awareness in that moment. You may be aware of this book in your hand, or my words if you are listening to the audio version of the book. Just notice. Notice where you are sitting or lying; notice any sounds that come into your awareness. If you find your mind wandering, perhaps to work, your children or your to-do list, come back to your breath. The breath you have now will always bring you back to where you are in each moment.

You can do this exercise at any moment that you find your mind wandering, or if you feel stressed or anxious. It can also be helpful to have a mantra such as 'breathing in and breathing out' to help focus your mind on your breathing.

If you haven't done a seated meditation before and you are considering it, think about what may be stopping you. Is it time? Is it confidence? Is it discomfort? Getting started can be easy. Begin with just five or ten minutes in the morning and you can increase that as you get more used to the practice. You don't have to sit on the floor; seated upright on a chair is fine. To help you could:

- Download an app and start with a guided meditation.
- Do a mindfulness course or eight-week challenge.

- Join a meditation group to meet others and get support.

Tip: Can you find somewhere in your home that is set aside for meditation. Perhaps a particular chair or cushion? This can help to create a regular habit.

Throughout the book you are going to discover areas of your life where you can introduce mindfulness, and each time you consciously bring yourself into stillness, you are creating a drop in the ocean of well-being.

Why meditation and mindfulness for menopause?

Physical changes take place in your brain from perimenopause right through to post-menopause. These can affect your emotional responses as well as being responsible for other recognisable aspects of perimenopause, such as having a foggy memory and feeling overwhelmed.

Caring for your mind is just as important as caring for your body during this time in your life. Regular meditation can help strengthen the part of your brain that regulates memory and emotions and help with planning and problem-solving. It can:

1. Help increase grey matter in your pre-frontal cortex, the area responsible for executive function, helping you to stay calmer when you would otherwise feel overwhelmed.
2. Increase cortical thickness in the hippocampus, which increases your capacity for learning and memory. This area of your brain is vulnerable to stress as well, so regular meditation and mindfulness can help to protect and nurture it.

3. Increase grey matter in your ACC, your anterior cingulate cortex. This is all about self-regulation and managing conflict. You know those moments when you find it hard to manage conflict as well as you may have done before, when patience is wearing thin, very thin? You can do something about that!

As you go through this book, you will learn more about your brain and how the different systems in your body benefit from reduced stress during menopause.

Integrating mindset approaches

Meditation, mindfulness and hypnosis can play a vital role in a new menopause care model. Rather than being an alternative therapy, they are complementary and an important inclusion in integrative approaches to menopause care, whether you are on medication or not. Using psychological tools can help empower you to be the wise mistress of your own well-being at all levels of existence.

At times that may be difficult. In fact, the thought of an 'empowering menopause' may be challenging in itself right now. Sometimes growth can demand a lot of you – but by acknowledging those challenges and being curious about them, you can open the door to great rewards. They give you an opportunity to arrive at a place where you feel as though you have more time to explore your choices, to try different things and to find out what feels right for you. You can learn to juggle the daily challenges you face, as well as the larger questions that emerge as part of menopause.

For me, more so than at every other stage in my life, meditation is the foundation for a mindful menopause. I can't think of a time when I've more deeply felt the importance of meditation in my life.

By learning and understanding both hypnosis and mindfulness you can apply different aspects of each of them at different stages and for different purposes. Sometimes I find mindfulness much easier to apply and, other times, hypnosis does the job perfectly. Understanding how to apply both can prepare you for whatever arises.

Summary

Both mindfulness and hypnosis can help you befriend different aspects of menopause. Meditation and mindfulness can help to improve memory, regulate emotions and reduce overwhelm. Hypnosis can help you to tackle day-to-day challenges, such as insomnia or motivation to exercise. Together they make a positive menopause possible.

2

Your Menopause Mindkit

Before the moon I am, what a woman is, a woman
of power, a woman's power, deeper than the roots
of trees, deeper than the roots of islands, older
than the Making, older than the moon.

Ursula K. Le Guin, *Tehanu*

I don't need to tell you that it's important to make time for
yourself and meet your own needs – you already know that.
When I give a presentation on self-care, stress reduction or
well-being, I know that everyone in the audience understands
the importance of self-care and I'm pretty sure that they know
what to do! But when I ask, 'Who regularly uses these tools?',
very few people will put their hands up.

So how can you integrate the tools into your life? The key is
to keep them simple – find what works for you and make it a
habit. During midlife and moving through menopause, life can
be busy and finding time for yourself can be tough. If you don't
already use reminders and plan all your time, including prioritising time set aside for you, start now.

*'What happened to my mind?! One day I went from hav-
ing a schedule in my head, able to juggle everything with*

aplomb, to not remembering appointments, forgetting to pay people, neglecting to pick up a shop. I had to learn how to use an online calendar that I could integrate with the rest of the family. Sometimes I still forget to put things in or look at reminders, but it's getting easier and I make sure that I schedule time in for me.'

Mandy

The hypnosis and mindfulness techniques in this book have a bit of magic in them, making the time you have feel more than it is. Instead of being crunched up and stressed in a particular window of time, you can calmly stretch yourself out and relax – it feels like an unburdening. It feels spacious. I use this time magic often in my life.

As you go through this life stage, being able to do this will become easier and easier. Like many women before you, you will start to feel your priorities shifting. You can move unapologetically from a place of self-*less* to one where you are becoming more self-*full*.

Gentle hypnosis exercises will guide you through goals, helping you to create healthy habits and let go of old patterns or unhelpful attitudes that limit your growth and potential to take on new experiences, or to follow your heart.

The mindfulness exercises you are going to learn will connect with your heart and encourage you to explore thoughts and feelings that arise, with curiosity and loving kindness. We'll also look at forgiveness and letting go in the context of different aspects of your life.

Many women I see put off using these tools – and that's because sometimes they can seem overwhelming. But they don't have to be. It can be a big step to embark on this journey or even go to a hypnotherapist to process something challenging, so I'm going to introduce you to small tools that are tailor-made for this stage in your life. Knowing you can make a difference in a matter of minutes is the trick to powering the positive changes that you want to make.

You may not want to sit in meditation every day for 15 minutes, but you can start with simple grounding exercises and daily moments of mindfulness. I encourage you to make this book your own, to discover the parts of it that really speak to you, the parts of it that you need to help you with certain experiences and the parts of it that get you through those difficult days.

What to know before you get started:

1. This book includes some quick fixes, but it will also help you create healthy habits and behaviours that support your well-being through midlife, menopause and beyond.
2. You will learn to create your own private space for reflection. These moments will help you re-evaluate the adjustments that may be happening and to look at them from a different and better perspective.
3. As you complete the exercises in this book and move forward, you may begin to notice that you are more responsive, calmer and more in control of what you are experiencing. Notice the days that are a joy, or when things flow and feel easy and you feel calmer. Write them down in your journal (we're going to get to that bit soon) so you can see progress.

The foundations we'll cover here are:

- Learning the value of acceptance
- The power of gratitude
- Journalling

- Meditation
- Self-hypnosis for change
- Affirmations
- Visualisations

Then throughout the book these will be crafted into tools and aligned with specific aspects that you may experience around your menopause.

Acceptance

With any life transition, acceptance matters. There are things that you want to change, and you can, but there will be things that you want to change and can't. For example, you can't change the fact that you are growing older or that your fertility cycle is shifting into a new phase. Some things won't matter to you and other things will be harder to let go of or come to accept.

All transitions are marked by challenges along the way. With attention, curiosity and the ability to let go of things you can't change, you can arrive at a place of acceptance. In acceptance there can be deep joy.

There are two aspects of menopause in relation to acceptance:

- Menopause-acceptance
- Self-acceptance

Menopause acceptance

It's happening! Pushing it away in your mind or trying to run away from it on the treadmill will not stop it from catching up with you. Menopause is inevitable. Your periods will stop, your body will age – it's all part of being human. Accepting it doesn't mean you have to like it; accepting it means that you recognise it for what it is. You can't second-guess when it will start or how long it will be for you, so I encourage you to stop thinking about it in that way.

Instead, you can throw your arms out wide and welcome it into your life and accept and work with it in a loving way. This will create the capacity for you to define how your relationship with perimenopause, and the time beyond it, is going to work so that your experience can be the best it can.

Self-acceptance

Not to be confused with self-worth, self-acceptance is when you are aware of and accept all aspects of yourself – the bits you love and the bits that you don't love so much. It can be hard to look at the aspects of your character or behaviour and say, 'You know what, I accept you for what you are' but if there is a time to do it, it is now! This transition, this new chapter in your life, is the last of three potential transitional milestones – adolescence, motherhood and menopause. It offers a meaningful and powerful exercise in self-exploration and love and compassion. If you want to accept the challenge, I promise you it's worth it!

There may be aspects of yourself that you find hard to accept or it may even be painful to acknowledge parts that are the result of the way that you have been treated by others in the past – perhaps your parents or others that you may have looked up to. Midlife can be the moment that you begin to see patterns clearly and accept those parts of you as a product of other people's expectations. This is a time to start living in your own energy, from a place a self-worth.

Throughout the book we are going to explore how this may manifest in many areas that challenge you during peri-menopause, allowing you to let go of the past and awaken you to your true power, unburdened by other people's stories and negative energy. I want this book to set you free.

Happiness and self-acceptance go hand in hand. In fact, your level of self-acceptance determines your level of happiness. The more self-acceptance you have, the more happiness you'll allow yourself to accept, receive and enjoy. In other words, you enjoy as much happiness as you believe you're worthy of.

Robert Holden, *Happiness Now!*

Menopause gives birth to a complex range of experiences, thoughts, feelings and emotions that may feel familiar to you. Sometimes those feelings may be intense or overwhelming; they may be born of grief and loss; they may be born of discomfort or loss of control; they may simply be there without you even knowing what they mean.

Often when a feeling is uncomfortable – whether it is physical or emotional – it is human nature to try to get rid of or avoid it. But what if you turned to the feeling with love and acceptance, despite the discomfort you may be experiencing. Imagine feelings like an energy; some are more powerful than others, but all of them are energy passing through. Acceptance is a way of turning towards this energy and being open to what it offers you. Like many things it is an experience.

It can take courage to lean into feelings that are difficult and uncomfortable, but by leaning into the discomfort and seeing it for what it is you give yourself permission to let go and release the emotional charge.

People who wade into discomfort and vulnerability and
tell the truth about their stories are the real badasses.

Dr Brené Brown, *Rising Strong*

Difficult feelings can be seen in their fullness and learned
from. They are your teachers during this transition – your personal menopause guides. The difficult feelings offer you an
opportunity for growth; an opportunity to become stronger and
wiser. This helps unite your dark and your light to find a place of
equanimity. When you accept all those feelings for what they
are, in any moment, you become aware of your own vulnerability, and you become more rooted in your sense of self.

Rooting yourself in this way helps create resilience in the
days, weeks and years to come.

A practice of acceptance is valuable at any stage of life, but
in particular around menopause. But what does it mean and
how can you use it?

Acceptance is action not inaction

I've had clients say to me, 'If I accept something but don't do
anything about it, then that's a weakness.' It's actually the
other way around. Choosing to do things that distract you
from those feelings is a form of avoidance.

It's a bit like pushing a rubber ball down in a bucket of water;
it will always bounce to the top. If an uncomfortable feeling
goes unacknowledged, it hangs around jumping up and down
like a child demanding attention, saying, 'Look at me, look at
me!' When you turn to look at the feeling – when you really see
and acknowledge it – it gently and lovingly stops demanding
your attention so vociferously. For example, accepting a feeling
such as anxiety is like accepting that it might rain when you put
your washing on the line. Like the rain, the anxiety won't be

there all the time; it will come and go and will sometimes happen at inconvenient times. Like the rain, you don't have to like or celebrate the anxiety – you can just notice it for what it is in that moment.

Acceptance is about bearing witness to difficult feelings whether they are emotional or physical. However uncomfortable they are you can choose to accept them, acknowledge them and let them go.

In a clinical setting, we work on very deep-seated emotions in a more intense way. If my client is working on accepting a particular feeling, I often see tears followed by a feeling of lightness. You may experience tears on tougher days, and that is okay – they are heart-opening tears. However, if you practise acceptance, you will mostly experience a gentle, growing feeling of ease in your everyday life.

Acceptance is a practice that you can learn to cultivate around menopause, and which can be a beautiful way to flourish and find joy in the years before and beyond it, helping you to find peace and joy.

EXERCISE 3: A PLACE OF EQUANIMITY

Put your hands in a prayer position. Now imagine that your right hand is the feeling pushing to be seen. Push it hard into your left hand and notice how the left hand automatically starts to resist. Keep trying to push the right hand into a resistant left hand and notice the tension in your body. Now just let the right hand soften where it is – allow it to be in that space – see where the left hand meets it gently. Imagine that left hand is your heart welcoming that feeling into a loving and tender space.

If you have overwhelming feelings, you can imagine your right hand as your feeling and your left hand as resistance or unconditional love. Breathing love into your left hand say, 'I see you with loving awareness.' Notice as your body softens.

Tip: The next time a strong emotion arises, you can experience the difference in pushing it away or practising acceptance. Take five minutes trying to push the feeling away, noting how many times the emotion bounces back again. Next notice the feeling or emotion, but observe it with acceptance and notice how it changes.

Keep practising these techniques until you learn to notice all feelings with love. They are all a part of who you are, and they are part of your story.

Gratitude

There is evidence to show that practising gratitude can improve sleep and your physical and mental health, which are fundamental to well-being in your midlife years and beyond. The findings show that people who practise gratitude are much more resilient, meaning that they bounce back better from stressful situations, build stronger social connections and have increased empathy. How incredible that something so simple that is available to everyone can have such a profound effect on our quality of life, especially in menopause.

As well as improving your well-being and your life experience, practising gratitude is proven to make physical changes to your brain. Grey matter is the outer layer of your brain and is part of your sensory nervous system, made mostly of neuronal cell bodies. At a time in your life when grey matter is sometimes shown to decline, practices such as gratitude can change the structure of your brain in a positive way. A 2008 study by the UCLA Mindful Awareness Research Center (MARC) showed that gratitude can maintain grey matter by activating neural pathways in several areas of the brain. A 2014 study showed that it can actually increase grey matter. Gratitude helps you become aware of things that help you feel positive and happy. As it does this it creates a pattern of gratitude, seeking out more of the same.

Gratitude may be something you practise already. You may even do it without thinking; it may come naturally to you or it may not. Often this is down to our own conditioning and life experience. Whether you do it or not, gratitude is a powerful tool that you can integrate easily into your daily life and that can make a subtle but meaningful difference to your experience of the time around menopause.

In times of upheaval, gratitude can support your brain when it's striving to find balance. It is being grateful not just for the big or unexpected joys that happen, but also for the small everyday things. I once had a conversation with a nun in which, bubbling over with joy and energy, she said, 'I am grateful that when I wake up I feel safe. I am grateful that I have clean water coming out of my tap. I am grateful that there is grass underneath my feet.'

As you unfold into this meaningful stage of your life, gratitude will connect you to a richness that may often pass you by. It will help you stop skating the surface of life and start noticing its depths, enriching even the most normal and seemingly mundane experiences. This heart-opening experience can add so much colour and joy to your life.

Throughout the book I'm going to invite you to use gratitude as a way to meet a particular challenge or experience. In the meantime, you can start to think about small daily changes that you can implement to introduce gratitude into your life.

Our attitude to gratitude often starts with language. Patterns of thought or unconscious behaviour are reflected in how you communicate with yourself and the world around you.

EXERCISE 4: THE LANGUAGE OF GRATITUDE

Just for this week, notice your language. How often a day do you say, 'I have to' or 'I've got to'. For example, 'I have to go shopping,' 'I've got to finish that project today,' 'I have to call Anna.' The words 'have to' and 'got to' imply it's an imposition, that it's a chore. Each time you hear yourself saying 'I have to' say 'I get to' instead. Notice what happens in that moment, and then over time as you begin to change your perspective of the world around you through the language of gratitude.

Put your journal to good use and write down things that have brought you joy or that you are grateful for. Be specific. For example, instead of 'I went to the cinema' write 'I got to go to the cinema and spend time with one of my children', or instead of 'I had lunch with a friend' write 'Today I got to spend time having a reflective lunch with Lisa'.

The power is often said to be in the giving not the receiving, so don't forget to externalise your gratitude. By showing other people that you are grateful for their input, their support or their kindness you build connectivity and community, both of which are really important as we go through the years before menopause and beyond. You can return a kindness with a thank you or a gesture, or you can pay it forward.

Expressing gratitude to others engenders a sense of well-being and calm in yourself.

Affirmations

Affirmations are positive statements that can help affirm or change a belief or help you fulfil a goal. For example, perhaps you want to connect with the confident part of you, or the motivated part of you. You can learn how to strengthen your inner resources to help you with a hot flush, or tap into your inner calm in those challenging moments such as when your teenage kids are flexing their hormones!

Studies show that affirmations can help foster resilience and help you in difficult situations, protect you against things that challenge your self-worth or integrity, reduce stress and help you achieve more at work. They do this by helping you to connect with and strengthen your values in a way that supports you.

Sometimes people interchange the words mantra with affirmations, but there is a very clear distinction – a mantra is a phrase, word or sound that has a spiritual meaning and is often sacred to a particular religion. An affirmation is secular and is a commonly used psychology tool that is used to encourage strength, positivity and well-being of body and mind.

Affirmations are one of the most powerful tools that I give to women. I didn't always think that way – they were the last rather than the first thing I would work with, but then I started to see amazing results. Now I spend time finding out what my clients' goals are, crafting the perfect set of affirmations and recording them to listen to every night. Affirmations are so simple, which makes them an incredibly versatile tool that you can use on a daily basis.

There is never a better time to use affirmations than during transitional times, such as perimenopause. When you are riding a tumult of emotion, perhaps feeling overwhelmed or finding it tough to focus on what you want, an affirmation can help ground you and refocus you. It's like a guide rope in the darkness that leads you to where you want to be in a subtle and gentle way. Sometimes it may feel as if an affirmation is not doing anything, but you have to trust that it will get you to where you want to be. If you really don't feel that an affirmation is helping you or it doesn't connect with your values, then stop. Like all the tools in the book it's about finding those that work for you.

Think about some of the messages you give yourself day to day. Are they kind, reassuring, encouraging, empowering, loving or positively affirming?

EXERCISE 5: AFFIRMING YOUR SELF-WORTH

This is an opportunity for you to write your own affirmations, ones that strengthen your connection to your mind and body in a loving way and counter the negative self-talk in your mind. Avoid words like 'try', 'should', 'might' and 'hope', because they create a get-out clause for the brain, and always write them as 'I' statements. For example:

'I am so emotional' becomes 'I am open-hearted and sensitive, able to freely express my emotions.'

'I am so disorganised' becomes 'I am spontaneous and go with the flow.'

Make sure that the quality is one that you align with. For example, if you are not or have never been spontaneous, that affirmation may not work for you. Connect with something that speaks to you, even if it needs a bit of dusting off! So, if you have become disorganised and would like to be less so, think, 'How have I been organised in the past? What part of me helps with getting organised?'

Step 1: Grab a pen and a piece of paper. Set a timer for 30 seconds. Now spontaneously write as many of what you consider to be the aspects of yourself that are stopping you enjoying this time of your life. Go!

Step 2: Now think of the values you have that will help you. *You can find a list of these on page 153 to help.*

Step 3: Now look at what you have written and write an affirmation that counteracts that statement using your values to guide you. Always remember to write it in the affirmative. Imagine you are writing an affirmation of worth to your best friend. If you can't do it all now, think about it and come back to it later. If you are surprised by how many negative messages you could write in that time, an affirmation along the lines of, 'Every day I speak kindly and gently to myself' may be one to add to the mix.

_____

_____

_____

_____

This is a tool you can come back to time and time again and adapt to whatever may be happening in your life, depending on how your internal landscape lies. I have a set of sticky notes and a pen in every room in the house so that I can write an affirmation in the moment and stick it up. I have affirmations on my computer screen, on the wall in the kitchen and by my bed!

Tip: You can also use affirmations to focus on the achievement of a goal, whether it's a micro-goal or long-term goal. For example, 'I am going to do a guided meditation every day this week before I go to sleep.'

Journalling

Diary-writing may have been part of your life as a child, you may have continued to keep a journal throughout your life, or you may dip in and out. It may be something that you have never tried. However you feel about journalling, now is a great time to try it.

Journalling for just 15 minutes three times a week over a 12-week period is evidenced to improve well-being. If you are experiencing anxiety, feel overwhelmed, or if you have a history of depression, journalling can be a very useful way of setting down your experiences.

Journalling takes on new meaning in the years leading up to menopause and beyond. Perimenopause is an adjustment over a longer period of time – having a yearly journal in which to set down your goals, to plan, to jot down the changes in your body, and how you feel can help to ground you. Your journal can act as a guide, a teacher, a companion and a listener. Each year, taking some time to reflect and look back on how far you have come can help the year ahead.

When you look back at the challenges you have overcome, you begin to realise that you can face others that arise.

To remember successful achievements reminds you that you are able to set yourself goals and work towards them successfully. To see goals that weren't completed can be a reminder that when things are in flux priorities may change and when that happens you are able to comfortably let go of things that aren't aligned with your purpose.

As you read this book, you may notice that thoughts pop up or feelings arise that you may not have considered before in much depth. This may in turn give rise to tumultuous dreams or moments when you reflect on past patterns of behaviour. Integrating the exercises in this book into your journal can help you week to week, month to month and year to year.

You could choose a journal that has sections set aside, or one that is blank. You can be as creative as you like and during the menopausal years you may find that your creativity starts to awaken. This often happens as your hormones start to shift, influencing the more creative right side of your brain.

Your journal could include:

- Drawings/paintings
- Collage
- Prose
- Poetry

If you really enjoy this, you could set up a menopause journalling group and get together with some of your friends so that you can chat, collage, laugh and encourage each other. The sense of community is something that will benefit you too.

As you continue through this book, you may want to journal about some of the tools you love or write down your Menopause Plan (see page 197).

The power of breath

There is a good reason why when someone is overwhelmed or has been in an accident, they are told to 'just breathe' or 'take a nice deep breath'. Noticing and changing the way that you breathe is a simple way to create a calm state of mind on a daily basis. Yet when life is trundling along and you're busy but not in the moment, how often do you stop and check in with your breath?

Breath is an integral part of your life; many different energetic disciplines rely on the breath, for example yoga and qigong – both of which work wonders for well-being during menopause. Breath gives life, and to breathe well expands our life force. There are many ancient practices around breath, upon which more modern practices are built that are used in studios and groups all over the Western world. In the past you may have been forgiven for calling some of these practices pseudo-science, but now science is finding ways to measure the impact of breath work on well-being.

The benefits of nostril breathing are of particular interest as we grow older, and especially during menopause. Remarkably your right and left nostril are connected to different systems in your body. When you breathe in through your left nostril, the breath triggers a rest and relaxation response, activating your soothing parasympathetic nervous system. Inhaling through the right nostril triggers your sympathetic nervous system, your fight-or-flight system. Studies show that alternate nostril breathing (see page 246) can soothe anxiety.

Often when we are busy, anxious or stressed, our breathing changes and we take shorter breaths that activate a state of alert, whereas a normal state of breathing would be an even breath in and an even breath out. This is sometimes called the 5:5 – 5 seconds in and 5 seconds out.

EXERCISE 6: BREATHING CHECK-IN

It's very easy to check how you are breathing at any given moment. Simply rest one hand just below your ribcage and one hand on your chest, close your eyes and notice which hand is moving more. Sit there for a few minutes and notice your breathing, the movement of your body. If the hand on

Breathing check-in

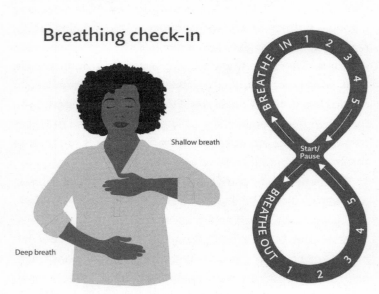

Shallow breath

Deep breath

BREATHE IN 1 2 3 4 5

Start/Pause

BREATHE OUT 5 4 3 2 1

your chest is moving more, see if you can switch to take deeper belly breaths so the hand under your ribcage moves more. Notice how your shoulders soften, and whether you feel calmer after doing that for a few minutes. Imagine how much better you would feel if you were checking in with yourself throughout the day at intervals to give your body an opportunity to find a comfortable, restorative breath. It's so simple, but it really works. As you connect with your breathing, you can begin to move to your Calm Breath (see next exercise), the breath that takes you into a state of relaxation.

🐾 EXERCISE 7: YOUR CALM BREATH

See page 9 for download information.

Once you have checked in with your breath and are breathing comfortably with an even breath in and out, you can start to take yourself to a deeper state of calm by lengthening your out-breath. This is a calming breath – or lengthening breath – which activates your soothing system and relaxes your body. Breathing in this way benefits your whole body (it can even lower your blood pressure) and improves your mood. I use numbers and words as a way to ground you in your breath (this is particularly helpful if your mind wanders), but also to create an anchor (see page 111). This means that the more you practise it, the quicker your body will respond to the words, '3-2-1, relax, relax, relax.'

When you feel anxious, turn to your Calm Breath:

1. Breathe in to the count of 3-2-1.
2. Breathe out to the words relax, relax, relax.

Choosing to practise the Calm Breath daily with focused attention for five minutes at a time can start to make a difference to your well-being overall, not just when you feel anxious. You can do it anywhere! At your desk, in a queue, while you are sitting in traffic – wherever you are and whatever you

Calm breath

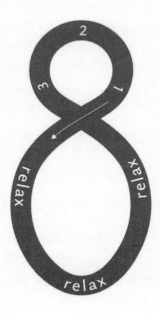

are doing, punctuating your day with a '3-2-1, relax, relax, relax' – your Calm Breath will start to support your body's adjustments in a very subtle and gentle way.

EXERCISE 8: YOUR MENO-PAUSE

I'm going to encourage you to take a Calm Breath at regular intervals throughout the book. Whenever you read or hear (if you are listening to this book on audio) the words Meno-Pause, stop, put one hand on your chest and the other one just below your ribs and tune into your breath. Say to yourself:

'This is my Meno-Pause.'

When you connect with your breath, start to move it to your Calm Breath and notice how the lengthening of your breath calms you and brings you into the present moment.

After you have finished the book, can you set yourself a target of at least five Meno-Pauses a day?

Tip: Print out (see page 9 for download link) and put up the illustration of a lengthening breath as a visual reminder of your Calm Breath. Unconsciously your mind will pick up on these calming cues and will switch you into your Calm Breath without you even thinking about it!

'I find time to be present
and aware.'

Self-hypnosis

Self-hypnosis is easy and safe to do – I teach it to all of my clients. By practising it, you can tweak the tools in this book to make them your own. If, however, you feel it's not for you, you can still do the exercises and visualisations without it.

You have everything you need within you to access a nourishing state of self-hypnosis with which you can create positive changes that will support you through perimenopause and beyond. Your inner drive, the heart of who you are, is to keep you safe and well – that will always come first. You will always come out of hypnosis if you need to – your brain is always on alert, even in a deep state of hypnosis.

If you are suddenly disturbed, it's not dissimilar to how someone would interrupt you when you are daydreaming.

Your alert system kicks in and you come back to the space you are in, fully alert. As you feel more and more comfortable with the visualisations and more familiar with the feelings associated with being in hypnosis, the easier it will be to discover the ability to do it yourself.

EXERCISE 9: HOW TO TAKE YOURSELF INTO HYPNOSIS

Find somewhere comfortable to sit or lie down – you may wish to refer to your retreat space on page 151. You may naturally feel cooler during hypnosis, which can be the added benefit of it, but keep a blanket to hand if you want to. You may still feel quite aware of your surroundings – it can feel a little like deep daydreaming. If you do self-hypnosis before bedtime, you may find that you drift into sleep afterwards, and that's fine. You can set an alarm if you want to be sure that you exit at a certain time, but pick a noise that will help you retain the feeling of calmness when you come out.

Step 1 – The Coin Relaxation

- Close your eyes and focus on your Calm Breath (see page 45) until you start to feel your shoulders and hands softening.
- Imagine you have a coin resting on the middle of your forehead.
- Keeping your eyes closed, imagine that you are looking at the coin, until your eyes strain a little as you roll your eyes upwards.
- Notice the coin in your mind, the weight, the details.
- When your eyes start to feel uncomfortable, relax into the feeling of comfort.

Step 2 – The Hypnosis Cloud

- Imagine that you are in a big soft cloud of self-hypnosis.
- Give that cloud a colour, and imagine your body sinking into that colour.
- Feeling a lightness and a sense of calm, as you breathe in your body becomes one with the cloud.
- If you were to hold your hand up to your face in your mind, it would be invisible.

Step 3 – The Deepener

- Count back from ten to one with each deep breath.
- Then just relax and use the visualisation tool you have chosen.

After self-hypnosis it may feel as if you have had a light nap, you may feel rested, you may feel a sense of heaviness as you come back into the room.

Tip: As you get more used to the feeling of self-hypnosis, you will be able to access that state very quickly and easily. You may find that you just need to close your eyes and skip to Step 2 – imagine being absorbed into your Hypnosis Cloud and counting down from ten to one. Throughout the book, I'll refer back to your Hypnosis Cloud.

Visualisation

In the years leading up to and beyond menopause, visualisation can really help, especially when you are using on-the-spot self-hypnosis. Once you've got the hang of it, it's quick, easy and intuitive. Using visualisation at this time of your life harnesses your imagination and it can be a fun tool. A lot of the success comes from believing that it works, and thankfully the research we have on this is extensive; the jury is no longer out and the link between imagining an outcome and your physical experience is known to be connected.

You can use visualisation on a regular basis, for short-term quick fixes or for longer-term goal-setting, such as a career change. It can even be used for changing your experience of something physical – for example, a self-hypnosis visualisation for tinnitus can turn unwanted sounds off in a matter of seconds.

When you use hypnotic visualisation, you light up a connection between two areas of the brain that directly connect the body and the mind. At the same time there is a decrease in activity in an area of the brain known as the salience network. This is the reasoning part of your brain that is working everything out. When this quietens down, it's like a superhighway is activated between your body and mind without any speed restrictions, traffic lights or police ready to stop and ask you why you're heading in the direction you are.

It means you can make changes without really thinking about it. When you want to change a habit, create a new one or change something physical that is happening in your body, it's the perfect tool.

EXERCISE 10: THE LEMON DROP TEST

Imagine holding a lemon drop sweet in your hand – notice the weight of it, imagine smelling it. Now imagine putting it in your mouth, and just keeping it there on your tongue. You may be noticing already that your mouth is starting to salivate. Now imagine it gently dissolving. You know that feeling of the fizz from a lemon drop? You may notice that as the sweet dissolves in your mouth, you start to swallow. When you are ready, imagine chewing it and then swallowing it. Notice how your mouth feels afterwards.

Your mind is powerful, and we know from research that by thought alone you can turn up pain, you can turn down pain, you can even turn it off. One of the keys to making a visualisation work for you is believing it can work.

'I am supporting and building the powerful connection between my body and mind.'

Visualisation is not always about seeing things in your mind either. I use the term visualisation because it's well known and identifiable, but it may help you to think of it as imagery – what you can imagine rather than what you can visualise.

Have you ever offered to 'kiss it better' when your child is hurt? Perhaps you've described your hot flush as a power surge or advised friends who are having a hot flush to 'imagine standing in a walk-in freezer!' Do you make a wish when you blow out candles on a cake? All of these are moments when you use visualisation in your everyday life without even thinking about it. This book and the visualisation tools within in are often coping strategies that feel very familiar because you use them all the time, without even thinking about it.

Throughout the book there are several types of visualisations that ask you to give feelings and emotions a colour, shape or image to help you to process change using your unconscious thoughts. Often this can change a physical feeling or an emotion quickly – it's the type of approach that works best with self-hypnosis.

The next exercise is a great visualisation. I refer to it often in the book to remind you that you can adopt it for a particular issue you may be having.

EXERCISE 11: MENOPAUSE HQ

Imagine that you have a Menopause HQ in your mind – your personal control room. Only you have access to it. This room can control thoughts and feelings. Throughout the book I'll refer back to your control room as it is one of the most powerful inbuilt tools that you have. It's a flexible visualisation you can use for anything. You can turn feelings or sensations up or down. You can have a shredder in it, and an incinerator to dispose of any unwanted thoughts or things that others have said that are lingering in your mind. It's really up to you!

1. Use your Calm Breath (see page 45) and your Hypnosis Cloud (see page 49) to go into a comfortable state of light hypnosis.
2. Imagine that you are standing in front of the door to your control room. What colour is the door? Notice the details.
3. Only you can unlock the door, which opens to a verbal password. What is that word?
4. Enter your room and notice how it is – there may be switches, dials and levers. Explore it and get to know it.

5. Notice how different aspects control different parts of your body or your thoughts.
6. For now, find the dial that turns down stress and the one that turns up calm.
7. Set both dials where you wish them to be.

Anytime that you want to use your control room, you can access it by thinking of the password. This will give you access to the enormous amount of inner resource that you have within you, just waiting to be unlocked.

I find it hard to visualise

If you find it hard to visualise, you are not alone. Some people find picturing an image really difficult while others find it easy. The reason for this is that we are all very different in how we process the world around us. Knowing how you unconsciously communicate can help you make the tools in this book your own. Off-the-shelf techniques are great, but when you take the visualisations in this book, moulding them into your own personal tools, they work at a much deeper level and they feel more congruent. Instead of thinking, 'This isn't working for me', think 'What would make this work for me?'.

Great hypnosis is about using your imagination well to change experiences, feelings, habits and behaviours. The Your Communication Style exercise will help to stimulate your imagination.

EXERCISE 12: YOUR COMMUNICATION STYLE

In this exercise I'm going to focus on these three senses:

- Feeling
- Seeing
- Hearing

I'd like you to pause and imagine a beach. There is sand underfoot, the sound of the sea, the feel of the wind against your skin. You can see a little boat bobbing on the waves, you can taste the salt in the air and feel the sun in your hair. Just close your eyes now and imagine those things, being aware of whether you can see things, feel them, hear them. Really immerse yourself in the experience in a way that feels comfortable for you. Sometimes it may be difficult to see the beach in full technicolour, but if you sit back and imagine your last happy holiday the details will come back very quickly.

Notice which senses are dominant. Do you feel the sea or see the sea? Can you feel a breeze on your skin, or do you hear the wind rustling in the trees?

Whenever you have trouble visualising, instead allow yourself to 'get a sense of it' in this way.

Your menopause goals

Throughout the book we are going to use goal-setting, both long-term goals and what I call micro-goals. Goal-setting is a great tool for getting things done when you feel tired and unmotivated, or a deadline is looming and you are procrastinating. Studies show that if you rehearse a goal in your mind, you are more likely to achieve it – for example, if you want to improve your exercise routine and motivate yourself to do more, simply visualise your goal. It's a motivation amplifier. You can also use goal-setting in the workplace to boost your confidence when anxiety is high, or to motivate yourself to complete a task.

Imagining your best, or desired, outcome can help to change your reactions and responses to opportunity around you. Whether it's an encouraging boost when you are tired, or a small daily task that you keep putting off, this technique is really effective.

Before we had the insight of brain imagery technology, no one was really sure why visualisation worked so well. Now we know that when someone imagines their goal, it affects the brain in a similar way to when the goal or action actually happens. One way of thinking about this is to imagine something that you don't like, or you want to get away from – you'll notice that you have a physical response; it may be just a subtle feeling of a tightening or contraction in your throat, chest or belly. For example, perhaps a particular food makes you feel queasy. If you were to imagine it right now in detail you may experience physically recoiling. If something comes to mind, give it a go.

Stop thinking about your brain as being in a fog and instead see it as shifting into a new way of thinking. Make use of the creativity that is awakening at this stage in your life. It's time to tap into that wildly imaginative and creative menopause mind. Become the architect of your own destiny by deciding how you want a particular event or experience to unfold.

You can choose to be an observer of how you wish to respond to a person at home or at work, or you can choose to observe yourself reacting in a different and better way to any physical experiences you have around menopause. You can choose to imagine yourself being joyful, capable, sleeping well or sticking to exercise goals, or maybe even starting your own business or a new hobby. It really is limitless!

When you create a goal-setting visualisation you become a participant and as you inhabit that experience with your imagination, your mind sets a course for that destination. This is a powerful step in deciding to make positive change in your life.

Let's start!

EXERCISE 13: GOALS FOR POSITIVE CHANGE

This five-minute exercise will feel a bit like daydreaming. Find somewhere quiet for it, where you won't be interrupted. Choose the best time of day for you, maybe before you get up or just before you go to sleep.

- Sit down or lie down and turn your attention to your breathing.
- Put one hand on your chest and one hand on your belly and simply notice your breathing.
- Then, as you feel your body moving into a state of calm or rest, you can begin.
- Think of something that you aspire to do over the next few days, months or years. It might be a weekly task you have been putting off or a big dream that you want to bring to life.

First be the creative director:

- Imagine you are creating a film of yourself doing this.

- Imagine all the steps to put it in place.
- Add detail – what do you need to do to make it happen?
- Make it how you wish it to be, with no barriers.
- If challenges arise, see yourself dealing with them.
- Go through the achievement.
- Notice the peace/joy/contentment you feel in achieving your goal.

You may need to go back and adjust a few elements. When you are really happy with it and the steps are clear in your head, become the participant.

Now be the participant:

- Now step into it, as if it's a film, and really experience it.
- Notice the steps you are taking.
- Notice how much easier those steps are when they are broken down.
- Notice how good you feel when you achieve it.
- When you get a strong feeling of achievement, lock it in your mind so you can come back to it quickly over and over again.

Tip: The more you imagine yourself achieving a particular goal, the closer you get to creating it in reality.

EXERCISE 14: GROUNDING YOURSELF

Throughout the book I'm going to give you prompts to ground yourself using this exercise. If you are feeling a bit distracted, lightheaded or discombobulated, it will help to bring you back into your body with a sense of stability and clarity. You can download it as an audio track (see page 9).

- Sit in a chair with your feet on the floor.
- Notice the soles of your feet on the ground.
- Notice your back resting against the chair.
- Take a deep breath in.
- Imagine that breath moving up from the ground through the soles of your feet, up through your body to the tip of your head, as if a thread of breath is gently tugging you upwards.
- Keep your jaw and arms soft.
- As you breathe out, feel the breath moving down through your body, down to where the soles of your feet meet the floor.
- Repeat the breath ten times. Continue to notice the rise and fall of the breath as it moves through your body.

'I am grounded, protected and connected.'

Summary

All of these tools are shown through research to support mental and physical well-being. As you read the book you will discover how to adapt them for your personal experience of menopause. The more you understand, the more you will be able to expand them beyond the content of the book to meet your specific needs. Their application is limitless, powerful and can be life-changing. Jump on board, and just give it a go!

PART 2

What's Going On?

Mapping Your Menopause

3

What is Menopause?

We delight in the beauty of the butterfly, but
rarely admit the changes it has gone through to
achieve that beauty.

Dr Maya Angelou

In this chapter we're going to lay the groundwork for the rest
of the book. It's not enough that I give you a set of tools and
say, 'Do these.' Knowing how your experience can be impacted
by what's happening both physically and culturally creates a
powerful foundation upon which to create change. Self-
efficacy is the belief in your ability to do something well.
Strong self-efficacy is built on knowledge of what is happening in your body. Something powerful happens when you
bring knowledge of menopause, shared experiences, tools
and techniques and physiological awareness together – you
unlock your self-efficacy, a deep-seated belief that you can
rock this menopause experience.

When does menopause begin?

How long is a piece of string?! Perimenopause leads up to your
day of menopause; it is a gradual change that often happens

Unlocking a calm and confident menopause

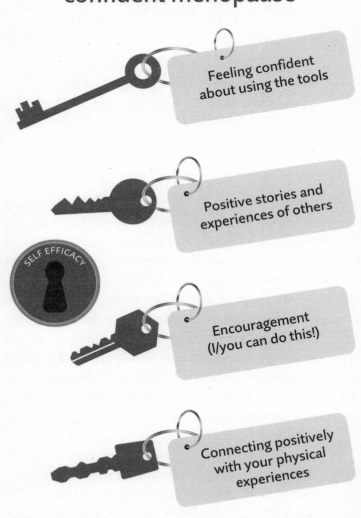

Feeling confident about using the tools

Positive stories and experiences of others

SELF EFFICACY

Encouragement (I/you can do this!)

Connecting positively with your physical experiences

earlier than we realise. I think very few people could tell you exactly when they started entering perimenopause. Most doctors agree that testing whether someone is perimenopausal can be a futile exercise as hormone levels can fluctuate so much from day to day, or even from hour to hour.

The best way to track your menopause is to really get attuned to your body and your own personal experience. Learning about your hormones and connecting with your body in a mindful way will support you to do this more intuitively.

'Every day my connection with my body grows stronger.'

Ethnicity and menopause

Everyone experiences a different timeline, but your ethnicity can influence your experience. For black or brown women, the average age for menopause is 49, whereas if you are white it is 51. The menopause transition may also last longer if you are black. Your experience can be influenced by cultural attitudes that are passed down. Physical experiences can also differ; black women may be more likely to experience vasomotor symptoms (see page 226) than white women. Japanese women are less likely to have hot flushes, but more likely to have joint issues. In many countries, inequalities in healthcare act as barriers for black or brown women and make it harder for them to receive the support they need. Learning about your ethnicity and menopause can help you to understand what's happening to your body and where you need support.

The average age for menopause is between 49 and 51, depending on your ethnicity (see box on previous page). Certain medical conditions can affect when menopause begins – for example, if you have Polycystic Ovary Syndrome (PCOS) your menopause may happen a bit later. The shifts and changes leading up to menopause can start years before when most women aren't aware that they are perimenopausal. It can be a feeling that you aren't yourself, perhaps being more irritable, impatient with children (more than usual) and fatigued. I've lost count of the number of clients, and friends, who say they feel 'as if they are going crazy'. Rest assured that you are not!

There is also early menopause, which is known as Premature Ovarian Insufficiency (POI). About 1 in 1,000 women experience menopause before they are 30 and it can be devastating for them. Many women I have spoken to say they didn't know what was happening or get the support they needed as menopause wasn't suspected by a healthcare provider. Support may also be limited, particularly as some don't wish to disclose this to friends or colleagues. The positive messages of transitioning into the wisdom years don't translate, yet the physical experiences can be profound and have lifelong consequences. Many of the techniques in the book will really help if you experience this – just skip over the age-related aspects.

Always remember that everyone is different; your experience won't be the same as anyone else's. Yes, there will be similarities, but you have an opportunity right now to learn about *your* menopause journey and to connect with your body, and to learn what's happening in your inner world.

Something to be celebrated

There has been an exciting move recently to celebrate the transitions in a woman's life in more profound ways – the onset of periods (the menarche) is something young children are more aware of. It is less hidden, less of a taboo and even celebrated. And now, menopause is making headlines, as a strong group of women show us how we can learn to embrace a shift into a potentially rich, vibrant and liberating stage of life.

Yet, menopause still exists largely within a biomedical model – this means focusing on the 'symptoms' and treating them with medicine, rather than seeing them as experiences, as natural physical and emotional shifts. We know more about artificial hormones and their impact on our body than we do about the natural shifts in our hormones and the impact of that on thoughts and feelings. Most women will have taken hormones in some form at some time in their life – perhaps as contraception, during birth, for fertility treatment or for other medical reasons. Hormones are a part of our lives.

In times of profound life transitions such as this, your well-being is far more complex than just the physical experience. Familiarising yourself with cultural, social and material aspects around midlife transitions can give you deeper insight into how to optimise your environment at home and at work. With the right insight and the right tools, you can feel calmer and more confident as you embark on your menopause transition.

The culture of menopause

Your experience can be affected by your expectation, and this is often shaped by your culture. It's not just about biological change, but also being alert to how the society in which you live views women of a menopausal age.

In cultures where youthfulness is aspirational, the word menopause is a firm reminder of ageing, and it's common to mourn the loss of youth. For those who want to stay as youthful as they can for as long as they can, there are of course always options. Cosmetic surgery is endemic; in some countries having Botox is like popping out for a cup of coffee. If you don't want to go under the knife, there are hair treatments to cover those pesky grey roots, moisturisers and ointments to stop crow's feet or sagging skin – so many creams! There are pants to pull in that troublesome spare tyre or squash you into a size smaller than you are – it's an industry that earns billions from perpetuating the beauty myth.

Not only are women faced with the very physical experience of ageing that seems to accelerate during perimenopause, but they are also on the receiving end of ageism in the workplace and the side-lining of older women.

'A friend of mine had said she had a sudden realisation she was invisible to the world. No one looked at you. If you are invisible you can do what you like as no one is looking at you! It was a bizarre confidence, a freedom. I put myself back into a place where I could see I would find a place of acceptance to feel okay. This approach gave me a lot of confidence.'

Bella

Conversely, in cultures where age is respected often the experience is different. For example, in some Asian cultures, fewer impactful symptoms of menopause are reported. This may have something to do with diet and genetics, but expectation also plays a very important role in experiences. One study showed that Indian women who had emigrated to the UK typically had experiences more consistent with white women living in the UK than Indian women living in India. This suggests that cultural influences have a significant role to play.

Why do we have menopause?

The reasons for menopause seem to be a bit of mystery. It is only experienced by humans, short-finned pilot whales and orca whales. For a long time, the assumption has been that we are no longer of any use once we have given birth to and raised our young; once we lose the ability to reproduce, we are surplus to evolutionary requirements. There is a school of thought that our role in species survival is redundant and that menopause is the beginning of the body's decline. Hang on, the truth may be a long way from that! Every woman supporting those around her, every mother or grandmother busy raising children and grandchildren knows that isn't true. Fortunately, new research suggests that menopause may happen for a very different reason.

Whales are now known to live in matriarchal societies, with the older female whales playing important roles in raising younger whales. They are often seen at the head of the pod, especially in times of need, guiding the other whales in their pod to food sources. It seems that their pods rely on their knowledge and experience. It's also assumed that menopause stops reproductive competition between mother and daughter, clearly defining their roles.

Like whales, women play an important role in raising grandchildren and contributing to the societies they live in. This is sometimes called the 'grandmother effect'.

The role of older women, the autumn queen and the crone has always been important: they are the storytellers, holders of knowledge, providers of herbs and wisdom. Our culture just seems to have forgotten this – and that menopause is our transition into this role, it's our rite of passage. Our autumn years and the time beyond even that, have been made into something to be feared when they should be something to be celebrated. It's an opportunity to mark your transition into a wiser woman, to fully embrace your menopause and prepare for a really positive experience as you move through this stage. Let's make it happen. Can you be part of the menopause revolution?

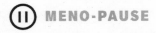 MENO·PAUSE

To fully embrace the menopause, it can help to understand at least the basics of what's happening so you can start to build those connections with your body and your mind.

What will I experience?

Factors that can influence your physical menopause experience are complex, but can include ethnicity (see page 65), the age when you started your periods, BMI, contraceptive medicine and genetics. It's not uncommon for you to have similarities with your mother's experience, or females on your mother's side – if you can talk to other women in your family about it, they may be able to give you some indicators.

You may have had, or be having, an early menopause (see page 66), or a medical menopause. This can happen if your ovaries are removed (oophorectomy) or if your ovaries and uterus are removed (hysterectomy). It could also be because of chemotherapy or radiation. You can also experience menopause if you have ovarian suppression therapy, though the ovaries usually start functioning again once treatment ends.

I really liked my uterus, the regulatory system and the balance. I have always been intuitive around my body. It felt like I had to suddenly, and with no choice, go through this series of doors and behind each door there was a pile of shit. I had to have cold turkey menopause as I couldn't take HRT.

Bernice

Often an early menopause runs in families, so if your grandmother and mother had one, then it may make it more likely for you. If they had a hysterectomy, it's worth knowing why they had one as this can teach you something about what you may expect. Every experience is different though, so use family history as a guide not a certainty; your lifestyle may be very different and we know that can be a factor in when you go through perimenopause.

'As I learn about my body, my mind aligns in restful balance.'

During your menopause transition, your brain, body and mind are constantly seeking to find balance – they are more closely linked than you may realise. It's a bit like the chicken and the egg: does the thought influence the experience, or the experience influence the thought? These are the questions I'm going to explore with you. In understanding the nature of your thoughts and feelings, you can learn to take control of the choice you have around your care, your lifestyle and your connections, all of which can contribute to a positive experience of menopause.

In Chapter 9 we are going to talk about your intentions for menopause, your Menopause Plan – you are going to learn tools that help you to advocate for yourself and feel completely comfortable and at ease discussing aspects of your life that you feel could be different and better.

EXERCISE 15: YOUR MIDLIFE DIARY

It's a really good idea to keep a diary of any symptoms that are impacting on your day-to-day life. Listen to your body. Whether you are experiencing hot flushes, changes to your periods, joint pain, irritability, anxiety, lack of sleep, note it down. Rate the symptom on a scale of 1–10, with 1 being of little impact and 10 being the highest impact.

Simply use a notebook or, better still, a pocket or online calendar via an app. These help you to keep an accurate timeline, with a place to write notes, giving you an overview of your experience and helping you to spot patterns, such as place or time of day. A record such as this is also helpful for your healthcare provider to be able to see the bigger picture.

Which stage are you in?

There are four very distinct menopausal stages that I see in my clients and each may need a slightly different approach. Read through to see which one fits you best.

Stage 1: Early perimenopause

You may be in your mid-40s, perhaps even younger, and starting to notice small changes. There may be a softness to your abdomen that is harder to shift at the gym. You may be a bit foggy in your thinking. You may surprise yourself with being more irritable and frustrated at things you may have tolerated in the past. There may be some hair thinning. You may start to get headaches before your period. The pattern of your periods may be changing, with a heavier menstrual flow.

Stage 2: In the thick of it

You may be in your late-40s to mid-50s, or maybe a bit younger. Your periods may obviously be more spaced apart than they used to be. If you have an app it may be telling you that your period is 'due sometime in the next two weeks' when it's been very regular before. Though it is worth knowing that some women's periods just go from being fairly regular to stopping completely. You may be experiencing your transition more intensely. There may be some hot flushes, you may notice that you skin is dryer and thinner, you may be experiencing some joint pain. You may feel unsettled in your marriage, in your friendships and notice heightened anxiety. At this point it is normal to feel as if it will never end . . . it will!

Stage 3: Coming out the other side

You will usually be mid-50s, or earlier. Your body has made significant adjustments and changes to get you to this stage. It may have been a smooth journey, or you may have had some bumps along the way. You may have created new habits and behaviours that helped you. When you have met the challenges around menopause, both emotionally and physically, you will find a new sense of balance and well-being. You can continue to grow into yourself, older and wiser than ever before.

Preparation is power!

This I cannot emphasise enough. If you are in your early 40s, or even late 30s, and you sense that you may be going through some changes listen to that little voice inside your head. That voice will become louder, but the sooner you listen to it the better. Even if you don't think you are perimenopausal, it's a good time to start to get into transition-supporting habits.

Many clients come to me for support when they are in the thick of perimenopause, or even when they are out the other side. I know that it would be easier to make the lifestyle changes they need to make, if they had begun preparing ten years sooner. This may sound like a long time, but hormone changes can start to happen ten years or more before the day of your menopause. The sooner you make the changes, the sooner they will make a difference to you and the more quickly your body and mind will benefit from them.

Think about the plans you make for other life transitions. If you were getting married, having a baby, going on holiday, or moving to a new house, you would put plans in place, wouldn't you? You may have done a lot of research and thought about what you do and don't want as part of this experience. I have never come across this concept for perimenopause.

Establishing habits and behaviours that optimise your physical and emotional health and well-being in the very early stages of perimenopause can be a game-changer. I have covered all of the things that you can do in this book, but it can be useful to use your menopause journal to jot down your goals.

These may relate to:

- Diet and nutrition
- Exercise
- Connections
- Emotional well-being

If you are in the thick of perimenopause and haven't prepared, then you are exactly where you need to be right now. The words in this book will rise up to meet you and will help guide you gently, as you learn to weave your menopause magic.

You are your hormones

I'm going to keep this section on hormones as brief as I can – I'm not going to tell you about pharmacological management or give you an encyclopaedic knowledge of your different hormones. Instead, I'm going to stick to what you need to know to piece together and understand the links between your body, your mind and the tools you are learning.

'You are your hormones' is something that you may have heard over the years; it's something that my mother kept telling me! And it is true that your hormones play a leading role in your well-being. Your first hormonal transition, during adolescence, may have triggered mood swings, acne break-outs and greasy hair. If you've had children and experienced pregnancy and birth, you may have been aware of hair thickening, breast changes and weight gain caused by hormonal changes. You may have had some postnatal anxiety and depression, and perhaps hair loss postnatally.

If you have experienced any of these physical changes in response to hormones in your past, you may be affected again during the time around menopause. Even if you haven't had experiences before of things like PMS, you may for the first time have periods marked by headaches and sore breasts. I see women who have never experienced anxiety who are absolutely at their wits' end, not knowing where it's coming from or how to deal with it.

Being curious about how you have responded to hormonal changes in the past can give you some clues as to what you might expect during your menopause transition and remind you of coping techniques that helped. In this way you can begin to make sense of what is happening and re-apply techniques you have used in the past to good effect.

EXERCISE 16: HORMONE HINDSIGHT

Can you look back and recognise hormonal changes at other transitional times in your life? Maybe adolescence, or, if you have had a child, think about pregnancy and postpartum. What have you learned? Just close your eyes for a moment and allow yourself to bring to mind your experience at other times when there have been significant hormonal shifts.

Was there an emotional theme? Were there physical aspects you found difficult? Spend a few moments noticing what comes to mind. Can you recall what you felt, which feelings were more prevalent for you? I want you to focus on no more than three, then write them down:

1. _____

2. _____

3. _____

Now think of three ways that helped you to feel better. What was your toolkit? Perhaps it was a person – maybe a counsellor or a friend – or something more practical, such as a breathing exercise or doing physical exercise?

1. _____

2. _____

3. _____

Meet your hormones

In times of hormonal flux, physical changes can be a fairly good barometer of change.

Menstrual cycles can help us to monitor hormonal changes. During pregnancy they stop, and, if breastfeeding, they may not become regular again until feeding ceases. Then during perimenopause as progesterone begins to drop, and your ovaries reduce their production of oestrogen, they change again.

Research on the role of hormones is growing all the time, not just on the use of Hormone Replacement Therapy (HRT) but complementary therapies such as mindfulness, hypnosis and Cognitive Behavioural Therapy (CBT) (see page 83), which can help with very specific experiences. From working with people during hormonal transitions such as pregnancy, motherhood and menopause, it's very clear to me that mindset tools can have a profound effect on experience.

Let's take a closer look at those hormones.

- Oestrogen
- Progesterone
- Testosterone
- LH and FSH
- Vitamin D
- Cortisol

Understanding how these hormones work can help you get to know your body and recognise the connection between an experience and a change in hormones, and help you be more informed when talking through your options with your healthcare provider.

Oestrogen: This hormone is produced by men and women, but females have much larger amounts of it. Oestrogen is responsible for the growth of the breasts, the lining in your womb and uterine tissue. In fact, all tissue in your body benefits from oestrogen, including your skin and brain. It also has a role in decreasing motility in the liver and digestive system and increases the absorption of nutrients. Bone density is also impacted by oestrogen, by helping reduce breakdown of bone. Oestrogen is largely seen to be a protective hormone.

There are three different types of oestrogen:

Oestrone E1: Around 50 per cent of oestrone is produced in the ovary, and the other 50 per cent comes from adipose fat and the adrenal glands, as it does in children and men. As the oestrogen introduced in our ovaries declines, we rely on our fat tissue and adrenal glands to produce this. Could that little bit of fat that creeps on during perimenopause be a form of protection?

It's also why, when preparing for menopause and beyond, adrenal support is so important, and this is something I'm going to talk about later as it's closely linked to our lifestyle, thoughts and feelings. We know surprisingly little about oestrone, its role and how its production is controlled.

A very recent study shows that this type of oestrogen is increasing, along with testosterone, in women over the age of 70. I would love to see a longitudinal study of this work being done in women from the age of 45 onwards. Is it possible that our bodies are making their own long-term adjustments to protect us as we age?

Oestradiol E2: This type of oestrogen, produced by the ovaries, is responsible for your periods and for reproduction. It has a role to play in increasing bone and cartilage density. As the ovaries start to produce less of this hormone, more common perimenopausal symptoms such as hot flushes, night sweats, restless sleep and hair thinning can occur. You may be surprised to learn that men also produce oestradiol; it is converted from testosterone and is important for sperm production. Like oestrone, it's also produced in small quantities by fat tissue, the brain and the walls of blood vessels.

Oestriol (E3): The production of E3 is triggered during pregnancy when the baby releases a chemical that helps its production in the placenta. E3 helps to grow the uterus and support a pregnancy.

Progesterone: This hormone comes primarily from the ovaries, but is produced in smaller quantities in the adrenal glands and brain tissue. Progesterone levels rise in the second half of the menstrual cycle, preparing the uterus for pregnancy by thickening the uterine wall. When the body sends a 'not pregnant' message, progesterone starts to decline triggering the shedding of the womb lining. During perimenopause, this is the first hormone to start rapidly changing – you may be aware of periods becoming a bit more irregular, cycles shortening and menstrual flow being very heavy. If you have PMS, you may notice that it's lasting longer, and if you haven't had PMS before you may notice some signs such as headaches, mood swings and breast tenderness for the first time.

Testosterone: Not many people talk about testosterone in relation to menopause, but it can matter for some women. It's known as an androgen and is produced in the ovaries and the adrenal glands. It's a hormone that peaks in your 20s and drops naturally as you age, but it drops acutely if you have had a surgical or medical menopause when its effects can be more noticeable.

Reduction in testosterone may impact on libido, reducing sexual interest, and may affect your experience of sex or reaching orgasm. Typically, in the UK this isn't prescribed on the NHS at the time of writing, but it is available privately both in the UK and other parts of the world.

LH and FSH: Let's not forget these two – Luteinising Hormone (LH) and Follicle Stimulating Hormone (FSH). FSH is the first to rise during your cycle – it's like a messenger that communicates between the brain and the ovaries saying, 'Now is the time to release your egg!' In perimenopause, as oestrogen levels being to fall, FSH rises to levels similar to early teens, working harder and harder to communicate with the ovaries. There is an interesting impact of raised FSH levels on the psychological aspects of perimenopause and beyond (see page 154) that many would see as positive.

Vitamin D: Okay, I'm going to throw this one in here as there is a lot of research coming out that tells us that Vitamin D is a hormone, not a vitamin. More accurately it's known as a pro-hormone. Remarkably the body only gets around 10 per cent of Vitamin D from diet; the rest of it is made by the body and produced in the kidneys. It's a really important hormone during perimenopause and beyond as it affects mood, bone health, brain health, the immune system and weight, all of which are impacted by declining oestrogen and progesterone. Research into Vitamin D is growing and a 2019 study found that healthy levels of Vitamin D may improve the experience.

If you live in the northern hemisphere, it is not unusual to have low levels of Vitamin D, as it is absorbed through the skin from exposure to sunlight. You may not absorb enough Vitamin D if your skin is covered with suncream or clothing when you are outside, or you simply do not spend enough time outdoors. Aim to get some sun exposure daily, within safe limits.

Cortisol: This stress hormone has a big role to play in perimenopause and is affected by other hormonal changes. Cortisol levels increase as we grow older and this can affect your circadian rhythm (your body clock), which is why sleep patterns may alter. Studies also show that a hot flush is usually followed by a rise in cortisol. I've included it here as cortisol is also sensitive to external stress and responds well to mind-body interventions.

Three steps to a smooth menopause

By becoming familiar with your hormones, and how your body responds to fluctuations and shifts, you will learn to create a deeper sense of connection with the transition you are going through. When you are connected, you learn to familiarise yourself with the experience you are having and manage it in the best way for you.

There are steps that you can take to improve your quality of life. I would always do step one first, as this is both preventative and can make a profound difference to your experience. If you find that this is not helping or that your quality of life or health is significantly affected, then move to the next step.

Step 1: Mindset-based therapies, exercise and diet
Step 2: Complementary therapies
Step 3: HRT and pharmacological interventions

Step 1: Throughout the book you will be introduced to different aspects of meditation, mindfulness and hypnosis that will improve symptoms such as hot flushes, help to regulate emotional health, and impact on lifestyle factors such as a healthy weight, sleep and your overall motivation. You may find that using these tools is enough to give you a good quality of life. I'm not saying that it will always be a breeze – there are bound to be tough moments – but they can go a long way to supporting you. I prefer women to start using these tools in their 40s if possible, so that they become easy and habitual – a part of who you are. The sooner you adapt to these, the more impact they will have. However, I have also worked with women in their late 50s who have found these tools just as powerful, so it is never too late to start.

Step 2: Remember that this is all about your quality of life, so if in addition to the Step 1 tools you find that you need a bit more support, consider using complementary therapies. For example, if you have joint pain, a sports massage can give some relief. Medical herbalism is popular and although the research evidence is mixed, anecdotally I know that many women have found this very helpful. Before purchasing or taking supplements, I recommend seeing someone who is trained in medical herbalism to help you find the right balance and supplements for you. Depending on other medication you are taking, there can be contraindications so always be careful. If you do buy off the shelf, opt for good-quality supplements from a well-known company.

Talking therapies can be used very successfully alongside medication you may be taking for a medical condition, or even alongside HRT. There are lots to choose from, such as Person-Centred Counselling, Cognitive Behavioural Therapy, Existential Therapy, Acceptance and Commitment Therapy (ACT) and hypnotherapy of course, which *is* my favourite! Look for a therapist that is registered either with the HCPC, CNHC or the BACP.

Whatever therapy you try, always shop around. Research shows that the rapport you have with your therapist can make a significant difference to your response.

Step 3: HRT stands for Hormone Replacement Therapy and is also referred to as MHT – Menopause Hormone Therapy. Over the past 20 years HRT has been mired in controversy, but that seems to be changing as more is learned about how it works and there is continuing research. What seems to be very important is that HRT needs to be balanced and tailored to the individual as much as possible. Dr Louise Newson, known as the Menopause Doctor, is a strong advocate of HRT and sees our bodies as hormone deficient in the same way that our bodies might be iron deficient, or Vitamin D deficient. She asks why would we happily take an iron supplement, but not a hormone supplement?

I'm not going to discuss the ins and outs of HRT here, but I strongly recommend that you do your research, if it is something that you are considering. I have included some excellent resources in the back of this book (see page 311), such as books, websites and podcasts, which explore HRT in depth, answering some of the common questions that arise. I have clients and friends who take HRT, but also some who choose not to take it or can't take it. They have all come to their decision based on what is right for them.

Managing choice

It can feel that control is taken away when you don't understand what is happening to your body, or how to respond to it in a way that is right for you. When making the right decision feels overwhelming and difficult, learn to navigate your options by using the three Ls:

1. **Leaning** into your experience
2. **Learning** about your experience
3. **Listening** to what your gut is telling you about the experience

Whether you take HRT or not is a very personal choice (or it may not be an option for you for medical reasons). Whatever you decide, remember it doesn't have to be all or nothing: pharmacological approaches to menopause can be combined with complementary medicine and self-help. For example, just because you take HRT doesn't mean you won't need to use tools to manage anxiety, boost your confidence or motivate you to exercise – there will always be challenging days and brilliant days. Life is still life. Always look at the big picture, ask your healthcare provider questions and remember you can always change your mind! Being part of the conversation enables you to choose your path.

'Menopause is just one part of my life.'

The gender health gap

The gender health gap is a term used to define the lack of health research that reflects women's experiences. This may be general research studies that are usually dominated by young men, through to the lack of studies into women's health, particularly in older age groups. More practice nurses are becoming specially trained in menopause, and I hope that this continues to improve, but as I write this many women go to their doctor as the first port of call and are given a wide range of treatments, including antidepressants. Perhaps we need menopause midwives?

'I was really desperate, suddenly I just couldn't cope, think straight or do anything. Carrying on like this was unthinkable – I wasn't sure how I would make it through another week of feeling so low. After seeing my doctor and talking to her about my experiences, I was given a progesterone gel. While on the gel, I did feel better even though it wasn't what I wanted. I used this time to learn more about perimenopause through podcasts, books and so on. I decided to stop taking the gel, much to the bemusement of my doctor . . . but before I did, I started to see a therapist. I felt more prepared and better equipped to follow what felt right for me. I'm not going to lie, some days are awful, but overall, I feel more connected with myself and it's not like I didn't have awful days other times of my life! Somehow I'm learning to manage them better and know myself better than before.'

Kirsty

EXERCISE 17: GETTING THE INFORMATION YOU NEED

Using this 'BRAIN' acronym is a great place to start when making a decision or talking to your healthcare provider about going on any sort of medication. You can start by using this format for getting the information you need from your doctor or nurse. Depending on where you live, there may even be a menopause clinic you can attend with nurses who are specially trained in supporting you.

Always remember that your doctor may not be able to answer all of your questions, so do more research if necessary. If your instinct is telling you that you haven't got what you need to make a decision, then you can get a second opinion.

BRAIN

B What are the **benefits** of the treatment for you?

R What are the **risks** of the treatment?

A Are there any other **alternatives**?

I What is your **intuition** telling you? What is the **indication** for this treatment or intervention?

N What would happen if you did **nothing**?

You can also see someone privately who specialises in menopause. There are more specialist menopause clinics being set up, which are privately run and offer an integrative approach.

Think of your hormones as a big troop of synchronised swimmers standing ready at the side of the pool – each hormone is one of the swimmers. If they all jump in together, they find their routine, they are attuned with each other. If one hormone jumps in too late, the routine may be a bit clumsy for a bit, but the others gently bring them back into the sequence. All sorts of external circumstances can disrupt the routine and all sorts of interventions can bring the dance back into formation.

If you have had a medical or a surgical menopause, it may be like removing oestrogen from the routine before the others have even got their swimming costumes on, and while everything is out of sync a substitute oestrogen jumps in the pool! Or one may have forgotten the routine, relying on the others to help bring them into the fold and find balance again.

The most important thing is to notice the swimmers, so that you can help guide them into the most fluid dance possible. Taking time to attune to your experience and using the BRAIN exercise will help you to explore approaches that work for you and for your changing hormones.

Summary

Your perimenopause is everything that revolves around the day of your menopause. You don't know when that is until 12 months after the event! Take control by learning about your hormones and the ways you can support your body and your mind. Your quality of life matters, your experience matters too. Explore your options, talk to people and educate yourself. Understanding what is happening and why it's happening will give you the confidence to calmly tune into your body and your experience.

4

Your Mind and Menopause

Yesterday I was clever, so I wanted to change the
world. Today I am wise, so I am changing myself.

Rumi

Although it may feel like it sometimes, be reassured that
you are *not* losing your mind and you are definitely not
the only woman who feels this way. You may have feelings not
dissimilar to when you were a teenager and your thinking may
be quite scattered or forgetful. Many women say that they
lose focus, and their mind seems to be ricocheting around –
trying to remember everything, but at the same time forgetting simple day-to-day appointments and tasks. It can be
maddening!

'Each day that passes it becomes
easier and easier to adapt to
the changes that are happening
in my life.'

Change starts in your brain and I'm going to show you ways to support these changes. You may have started to doubt your brain's capacity to work in your best interests, especially during perimenopause, so I want you to understand how smart it can be.

Remember that it's not the brain you were born with. As you have grown older and wiser, your brain has become enriched with memories and experiences. It's true that experiences beyond your control – whether those are from childhood, adulthood, trauma or work – can shape your brain, but this also means that you can learn to recognise, choose and create experiences that can support you.

When I first learned of aspects of perimenopause that I was able to manage more comfortably through tools such as hypnosis and mindfulness, I felt really excited to discover that I was far more in control than I had ever imagined. This is something that I want you to experience as you read this book. You are going to learn that your brain is an incredible organ, complex and unusual, with an active role to play during this time of your life. Imagine it as a control centre that you are in charge of – see the control room visualisation on page 53.

(II) MENO-PAUSE

It has taken far longer than it should to start to understand the female brain in relation to the menopause – typically, women know much less about their health, both individually and collectively, because of the gender health gap (see page 85). These research gaps mean that we largely fumble our way through, without the knowledge that we need to be able to support the changes that are happening in our body and brain. However, thanks to a leading group of researchers globally this is starting to change. We are learning how our brains change, and the impact that these changes can have on us.

The very same research that's teaching us about the impact of hormonal changes on our bodies, is also giving us an opportunity to learn approaches that support our bodies and our brains. Rather than thinking about all the negative aspects of perimenopause and beyond, I want you to start to think about the positive aspects. Researchers are giving you a golden opportunity to learn to adapt to, if not eliminate, some of the experiences you may be having, as well as how you can take better care of yourself for long-term health. Much of it starts in your brain.

Your brain is working hard at navigating you through this time of adjustment, and you have everything you need within you to support yourself.

What the ?!?@ is going on?

The focus on menopause is always hormones. 'It's my hormones!' is something that you will often hear from friends, colleagues and in ubiquitous menopause memes in the media to excuse clumsy behaviour, forgotten appointments or angry outbursts. Yes, hormones play a vital role, but so does your brain. As you go through perimenopause, your brain loses some of the neuro-protective benefits of oestrogen, but you don't have to resign yourself to a life of foggy thinking. Your brain is like a computer that is reorganising itself to be as efficient as possible for this next stage of your life. While it's reorganising you just have to find your way around and have patience. The fogginess will pass.

'I am resourceful and resilient; I will
find the way that is right for me.'

Despite hormone-related fogginess during perimenopause, and in other stages of your life, you've juggled and
you've hustled. You *are* resourceful. Think of those times in
your life when you have found a way through something
impossible, or the creative methods you employ to manage
the day-to-day balancing act of juggling home and work. You
probably do this while not even thinking about it consciously
(if you can't remember a time right now, you will soon after
you have read this). Never underestimate what you are capable of or allow other people to limit your potential.

During perimenopause it can be helpful to create grounding
habits and rituals that give you balance. Recognition and acceptance that this is a normal part of life as it unfolds, can help you
to adapt your daily schedule in a way that works for you.

🎧 EXERCISE 18: STARTING YOUR DAY WITH JOY

See page 9 for download link.

Grounding yourself in the morning means you can start
your day with a connected body and mind, which sets a
calm tone for the rest of the day. You may be someone who
is very alert in the mornings, or you may be someone who
needs a bit of caffeine to get the wheels in motion. However you begin the day, this exercise will benefit you. It only
takes five minutes and you can do it sitting or lying down. It
involves a breathing technique and a gathering in of
energy, so that you feel focused and strong instead of

scattered and disrupted in your thoughts and actions. To set an intention to start the day in this way is a powerful message to your mind that you are ready for business!

Tip: Learn how to use voice recorders for notes, diaries and so on. Many women have what they call The List. If you have managed up until now without one and have it all in your head, carry on, but if you have a large family and are finding it difficult to juggle the diaries for everyone now may be the time to start one.

Your menopausal brain

Your brain is an amazing organ with billions of connections that help you function day to day. It is made up of different sections that all have a role to play in how you react and respond to your internal and external world. They all communicate with each other using an elaborate communications network of neurons. Your brain adapts and changes at different stages of your life to help optimise your well-being. This ability to change is called neuroplasticity. Research shows that we have plasticity in our brains well into our 90s and probably beyond.

It's well known that Black Cab drivers, who have to memorise the streets of London, have benefitted from brain plasticity – their brains are wired to be enlarged in the area that's responsible for spatial representation. There are so many case studies of the brain's ability to rewire and use different areas of the brain if there is brain injury. It's this ability to rewire and strengthen the brain that you can really benefit from during perimenopause, and even beyond menopause. You've probably heard the phrase 'neurons that fire together, wire together'. It's never truer than now.

Research shows that grey matter starts to decline during perimenopause and beyond, and this is one of many negative take-home midlife messages that women are sold. In truth, grey matter starts to decline for everyone, no matter what gender, as they grow older. Women seem to be at greater risk of Alzheimer's, but despite the gender health gap we are starting to learn why this is and what is preventative. While what you eat, and how much you exercise are known to be important factors, we need to talk more about continuous learning and the role of social support – communication and community involvement. It's not just something that we should think about in relation to elderly people in retirement homes; it's something we should all aspire to make space in our lives for, especially from midlife onwards, as it's protective and regenerative. Embedding good habits in your life from perimenopause onwards will help your mind as well as your body.

I first came across the 'Nun Study', led by a researcher called David Snowdon, a few years ago. Snowdon wanted to understand what caused some people's brains to stay healthy while others deteriorated. A group of nuns in Minnesota agreed to leave their brains to the study when they died, and since then it has grown to over 600 nuns all over the world. Snowdon has access to all their records from a young age, and because they have very specific lifestyles it makes for interesting data.

It's believed that we build up a 'cognitive bank'; our knowledge, use of language and how engaged we are with learning can all contribute to this. The nuns in this study are socially active within the local community in many different ways. This constant learning and the frequent 'deposits' in their cognitive bank, help the brain rewire in some parts while other parts still become inactive. Keeping your mind connected and knowledgeable keeps you alert and healthy.

One of the cases in the 'Nun Study' was Sister Mary who died aged 101. She showed no sign of cognitive decline, yet her brain showed significant degeneration in line with advanced dementia. She had questioned whether her doctor was giving her medicine to keep her alive, but her doctor replied, 'It's your attitude!' Snowdon said that 'she was alert and involved . . . in the present moment with all her heart and soul.'

EXERCISE 19: LOOK AFTER YOUR BRAIN HEALTH

The ideas here will help to offset any natural decline that happens during ageing and help protect your brain as oestrogen drops.

1. **Learn a new skill or do something that makes you think:** Learn a musical instrument, a new sport, or study something that interests you. Challenge your mind and keep going. You can wire those neurons, but firing them over and over again will make them more established.

2. **Learn or improve a different language:** If you are multilingual and use more than one language on a regular basis, it's evidenced to reduce cognitive decline. Consider watching films or listening to the radio in a different language, perhaps one that you learned at school.

3. **Stay connected:** Socialise with friends, go out, volunteer in your community or at work. University of the 3rd age (U3A) is an organisation that creates opportunities to do something new. It's run by volunteers, so you can always volunteer as well!

4. **Movement and exercise:** Regular movement supports the development of new neural networks.

5. **Nutrition:** Omega-3 and Omega-6, found in oily fish, nuts, seeds – such as flaxseed – are shown to play a role in protecting brain function. Some foods also have a role in gut health, which can help lower inflammation, helping to maintain healthy neural pathways.

6. **Your mind:** Mindfulness, meditation and hypnosis are shown to reduce stress, which has an anti-inflammatory response and huge benefits for your cognitive health.

I'm going to cover points 1–5 later in the book and give you some hypnosis and mindfulness tools that will help motivate and encourage you to integrate these simple habits into your life, so that they become sustainable moving forward.

For now, I'm going to expand on point 6 – your mind and menopause.

Mind over menopause

Attitude may not be *the* only fix, but it goes a long way towards changing your day-to-day experience. With optimism, positivity, a willingness to accept and let things go with lightness of heart, love and the courage to try new things, you can create formidable resilience that will help you on even the toughest days.

1. **Meditation and hypnosis increase blood flow to the brain, which can protect against neurodegeneration:** By increasing blood flow to the brain, keeping fit and eating healthily, you care for your telomeres, which can be found at the end of every strand of your

DNA – imagine them as the protective bit of plastic on a shoelace. Stress, reduction in oestrogen and obesity are three factors that impact the health of telomeres, which can be seen as your internal body clock.

Lifestyle choices can also affect the health of your telomeres. Meditation and hypnosis are known to support healthy telomeres. In fact, one study showed there was a 43 per cent improvement in the health of telomeres following a regular practice of Kirtan Kriya meditation, a multisensory meditation that is shown to increase blood flow to the brain and protect against neurodegeneration. In Eastern tradition this is understood to bring your body, mind and emotions into balance. Try to set yourself the challenge of doing this for a week. It's a very popular meditation and there are many videos with verbal guidance on YouTube. Refer to the resources section (see page 312) if you want to know my favourite.

2. **Meditation helps to maintain and even increase grey matter:** Your cortex, which makes up the outer part of your brain, starts to thin as you age. As this is associated with memory and decision-making, it's definitely a part of the brain worth taking care of. Imagery studies show that meditation can reduce the decline of grey matter in the cortex, while other studies show that it can increase grey matter density in the area of the brain known as the hippocampus, which is important for learning and memory.

3. **Both meditation and hypnosis improve concentration:** As the perimenopause brain starts to reorganise itself, there may be times when you find it difficult to focus on the things that you have to do. Mind-wandering is something that most women will testify to at this stage in their lives. You can improve your ability to focus by using meditation – and a very specific meditation that

focuses on an object for a certain length of time (see the exercise below) can improve your ability to focus attention in daily life.

EXERCISE 20: CONCENTRATION CANDLE

This very simple meditation helps to improve concentration and memory. It's easier to do if your space is dimly lit and the temperature is comfortable. Sit in an upright position with the lit candle positioned so that you can look at it comfortably. Just stare at the candle, noticing every detail; allow all of your attention to remain focused on it. It's normal for your eyes to water if they feel dry, as is sometimes the case. If this happens, blink a few times and then come back to the exercise.

It is normal for your mind and your eyes to feel like wandering. As you continue, that desire will fade. Just notice and then focus back on the candle. A simple way to really connect with this meditation is to imagine breathing the candle in and out.

The experience can be very peaceful. As sensory input from elsewhere in the room starts to fade, you become more connected with the candle and your attention is focused, while your mind is still. If you move and bring in other sensory input, you will notice the difference between being in that state of focused attention and stillness compared with the feeling of having lots of sensory input.

When you have finished, remember to blow the candle out. Sit peacefully for a few minutes as you reorientate and come back into full sensory awareness.

Hypnosis is also evidenced to improve concentration and memory by slowing brainwaves down. Regular use of hypnosis, either self-hypnosis (see page 48) or listening to a hypnosis download, will help improve your memory. Happily, any of the downloads you listen to as part of this book, whether it's letting go of the day, or well-being, have the marvellous side-effect of improved memory.

4. **Meditation and hypnosis can reduce cortisol levels:** Cortisol (see page 81) is one of your stress hormones. We all need a little of this, but in times of stress and during perimenopause cortisol levels are something that you need to keep on top of as best you can. High cortisol can impact on progesterone, having both a physiological and psychological effect. You'll learn more about this link in Chapter 5.

5. **Mindfulness and meditation combat brain shrinkage:** The real name for this is atrophy, but it's used so much in relation to menopause as a descriptive term, suggesting lack, that from this moment I'm not going to use it! Throughout perimenopause, and as oestrogen declines, the brain naturally starts to get smaller. Sounds awful doesn't it? But Sister Mary (see page 95) had a brain that only weighed 870g when she died, a brain weight that correlated with severe cognitive decline. The average brain weight of someone aged 65 is around 1.2kg. She was still alert and sharp when she died. A busy small brain can fire well – it's live-wired, and re-wired over and over again because it's always active. Not only do mindfulness and meditation optimise healing in the brain and reduce stress, but hypnosis can help motivate, encourage and give you confidence to try new things, to meet new people, and to test the boundaries of life in a way that feels invigorating and enlivening.

Tip: Hypnosis is all about re-framing so instead of thinking brain atrophy, think 'I have a trophy brain.'

Making menopause waves

Let's talk brainwaves. If your brain is busy all the time, in a gamma or a beta state, it's working hard. Brainwaves indicate different levels of brain activity, and one of the skills your brain is going to have to learn during perimenopause is how to rest, to slow the waves down and allow them to lull you into a state of calm. A restless mind can upset hormones and have an impact, not just on your physical experience but also on your thoughts and feelings.

Meditation, mindfulness and hypnosis all have the remarkable ability to change your brainwave activity and help you to rest your mind in a restorative way. Your brain is doing some heavy lifting and needs a breather every now and again. By using these tools, you are actively choosing to slow your brainwaves down and quieten that voice in your head.

They also protect you against fatigue and stress, which can exacerbate any physical aspects, particularly hot flushes, sleep disruptions and weight gain.

EXERCISE 21: MINDFUL MOMENT

Taking a Mindful Moment at regular intervals throughout the day can make you feel calmer, and more creative. If you have a busy life, balancing home and work, set a reminder on your phone to stop and connect to your body, slow your brainwaves down and give your brain a breather.

Your brainwaves

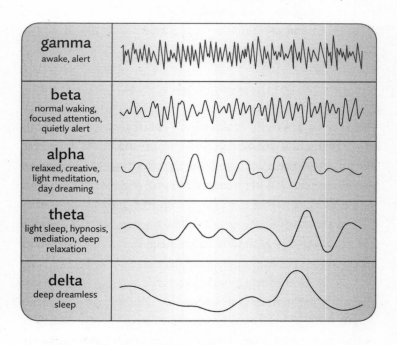

gamma awake, alert	
beta normal waking, focused attention, quietly alert	
alpha relaxed, creative, light meditation, day dreaming	
theta light sleep, hypnosis, mediation, deep relaxation	
delta deep dreamless sleep	

1. Wherever you are – perhaps sitting at your desk, stuck in traffic, waiting for the kettle to boil – notice your breath.
2. Keep noticing your breath, breathing in and breathing out.
3. Notice where your feet meet the ground.
4. Notice any sounds that come into your environment, name them and let them go.
5. If your mind wanders come back to your breath, breathing in and breathing out.
6. Continue for a minute, or longer.

Your menopause zone

These years are a rite of passage, a quest that turns inwards towards the heart of who you are. As on any quest your eyes need to be on the road ahead, alert to interlopers that threaten to distract you. You need to be prepared and well equipped to tackle challenges that can often be opportunities in disguise.

You just don't know how it will be for you, so take one day at a time staying grounded in your menopause zone where you can rest and strengthen your mind.

You can find solace, power, rest, love and joy in this place. These are the moments when you are centred, grounded and connected with your experience. Unwavering in your strength, even when a part of you doubts that you are strong enough, or wise enough, or . . . just enough.

When you are in your menopause zone, you exist where you are, in body and mind. Whether there are distractions, upsets, difficult experiences, losses or grief, you can ground yourself in your zone – your redoubt.

If at any time you are feeling overwhelmed, stressed, pressured, uncomfortable or angry, use your Calm Breath (see page 45) to ground yourself in your zone.

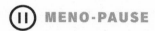 **MENO-PAUSE**

Remember, these difficult moments are also the transformative moments, the moments when you make a choice to go deeper, and to grow stronger and wiser. When everything feels like it's unmanageable and you choose to connect with what is happening in that moment, you are deepening your commitment to a growth experience.

Bubble of calm

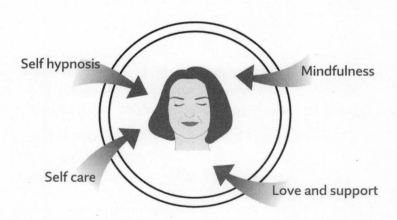

EXERCISE 22: IT'S ELEMENTAL

To ground yourself in your zone quickly and easily, it helps to connect with one of the elements. You may gravitate to a particular element – read this list and let your intuition guide you to which one is most connecting for you.

Earth: Notice where you are standing, the ground underfoot, your connection it. Notice the details of where your feet meet the ground. Sitting in the roots of a tree can be grounding too. Perhaps it's time to become a tree-hugger!

Air: If you are outside, notice the wind on your skin, the temperature, the leaves moving in the trees. Notice the air. Notice your breath, the coolness of the air as you breathe in and the warmth of the air as you breathe out.

Water: If you are at home, place your hands beneath a running tap. If it's raining, stand in the rain, or if you are near moving water connect with the sound. Listening to a download of running water, the rain, or the sound of the ocean can help. It's no coincidence that many people retire to the sea!

Fire: You can stand in the sunshine, or in winter next to a firepit or bonfire. Even lighting a candle can help ground you in fire energy – see the candle meditation on page 98.

Hypnosis boost: If you can't get outside or can't connect with the energy you have chosen, close your eyes and imagine being near water, or fire, or earth, or out in the fresh air. Really build the image of being near the element through your senses.

Tip: Keep a grounding pebble in your pocket. If you go on a mindful walk (see page 281), find pebbles that appeal to you and put them in the pockets of clothes and coats. Then when you are out you can hold the stone, to connect and ground yourself in that moment.

Summary

Be kind to your brain as it stealthily navigates the ebb and flow of a different hormonal rhythm. Be its protector by choosing healthy habits, have a go at new things – tap into that growing confidence within you. Recognise the times when you are tired and overwhelmed as a time for rest. Use your mindful moments, ride the waves of emotion and experience, and get used to grounding yourself in your menopause zone.

5

Fearless Menopause

When I get frustrated, all of that upsets my heart,
and it's not worth it, so I just say, 'I love my thoughts.

Ram Dass

As you work through this book, you will become more and more aware of how unconscious thoughts can influence your experience and how to change them. Being able to live in your experience fearlessly will help you see beyond the fog of perimenopause, learning how to apply techniques in the moments you need them most.

In this chapter we are going to get under the skin of fear and stress to lessen them. This will help you to unlock your true power as you move through this stage in your life and improve your experience of menopause.

Let's dive in!

Anxiety or fear?

Before we dig a bit deeper into anxiety and fear, it helps to understand how they are different. Anxiety is the fear of something that may never happen. Fear is an in-the-moment response to something that is happening. Though anxiety and fear are different, they elicit similar physical responses:

- Increased heart rate
- Shorter, shallower breaths
- Foggy thinking
- Feeling lightheaded
- Sweaty palms

Intense anxiety can lead to a panic attack – as breaths become shallower, it can be harder and harder to take a breath. This is not a usual part of the perimenopause, though someone is more likely to experience it if they have a history of anxiety or postnatal depression. It's more common to experience increased feelings of anxiety about aspects of daily life. Sometimes anxiety can be associated with something very specific or it can be what is known as free-floating anxiety or generalised anxiety disorder (GAD).

As you learn about your physical responses to expectations and experiences of the perimenopause, I want you to consider whether something is anxiety or fear. If you are not at risk in that moment, it's anxiety, and the power to alter your response to that feeling belongs to you. You can change how you feel. In Chapter 12 on tackling anxiety, you will learn more practical day-to-day tools to help reduce anxiety and increase calm in your daily life.

Fear of mortality

I am not including fear of mortality to frighten you. If you feel that lurch in your stomach when reading this, it means that the fear is there anyway, under the surface. If you want to have a fearless and confident menopause, this may be something that you need to spend time understanding.

Unlike men, women have very clear markers of their stages through life – motherhood and menopause are two of the most intense. There may be grief for lost opportunities, paths that weren't taken, you may be worried about time passing or fear that time is running out. People often comment that time moves faster as we age. Although many things in our lives are unpredictable, the one thing that is predictable is our own mortality, and although that may seem like a negative way of thinking, it's an irrefutable reality. We come from nothing to something and back to nothing again. We are impermanent. This realisation can come in waves at this stage in your life, so allow those waves to pass through, just notice them and then come back to the moment you are in.

Being in a state of fear is to be living in a trance state – it's a form of hypnosis. When you are not in the present moment, and alive to what is happening, you miss it. Think of a car journey that you are very familiar with. You get in your car, you turn the engine on, perhaps have the music on in the background. You are busy with so many things to do, your thoughts may be wandering to your to-do list, you may be thinking about your children. Absolutely consumed by thoughts, you still manage to drive home and when you park up you might think, 'Wow that went fast' and you may not even remember the journey. The route is so familiar, your unconscious was able to drive it – it guides you through your day-to-day life.

Life can be like this. Time can pass quickly while we don't notice it passing. Instead of seeing mortality as something to be feared, use it as a reminder to live fully in the present. If you are looking back to the past and into the future, you are not living right now in this moment.

'I use my time wisely and joyfully witness all that life offers in this moment.'

To live a fulfilled life is to literally fill those moments up with meaningful experiences – to fill yourself up with experiences you have to be in them. It may be as simple as noticing a flower that has unfurled in your garden or the cosy feeling of your partner, child, or grandchild curled up against you on the sofa. Or it might be going on an incredible outing or holiday. When you stop living outside the moment and instead are fully in it, you may discover that time feels more expansive than ever.

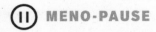 **MENO·PAUSE**

At my age, in this still hierarchical time, people often ask me if I'm 'passing the torch'. I explain that I'm keeping my torch, thank you very much – and I'm using it to light the torches of others.

Gloria Steinem

In truth we never know when our last day is, so let go of the fear of loss and find joy and happiness in every day; make every day matter. The very nature of your existence is extraordinary – your thoughts, your body, the leaves, the rain, the sun, the plants, any mini-humans you made, the ground underneath your feet, the stars above your head. It's all incredible isn't it! Sometimes just stop and reflect on how this is and say the words . . .

'Breathe, you are alive.'

Thich Nhat Hanh

Coming back into the moment by connecting with your immediate environment is soothing and stabilising. The following exercise is one that I personally use a lot when I am feeling overwhelmed.

EXERCISE 23: THE SPOTLIGHT

Imagine that your mind is like a spotlight that can only focus on one thing at a time. Your spotlight may be moving around really quickly if you are balancing lots of different things, unable to really be present in the moment you are in. This exercise brings you back into the moment, and also rests an anxious mind. Done regularly you can train your mind to rest in the moment you are in.

You are going to use three of your senses: seeing, hearing and feeling.

- You can start with your eyes open or closed or close them at any point during the exercise. If you have them closed, just notice what you can hear and feel.
- Breathe in and breathe out until your shoulders are softening.
- If you find your mind wandering, come back to your breath.
- Use the affirmation 'breathing in and breathing out' in your mind as your anchor.
- Notice what comes into your attention in any moment.
- Notice what you can see (if your eyes are open).
- Notice what you can feel – both feelings and touch.

- Notice what you can hear.
- Keep continuing to notice what you notice and name it – for example, traffic, voices, hunger, frustration, silence.
- If your mind wanders, come back to your anchor, 'breathing in and breathing out'.
- See if you can do this for five minutes a day at least. It's a great exercise for when you are filling the car up with fuel, or waiting in a queue.

Tip: You can use this as an exercise in focused attention in your garden for ten minutes a day. Noticing the wind, flowers, plants, insects – you'll also benefit from Vitamin D exposure!

Your spotlight

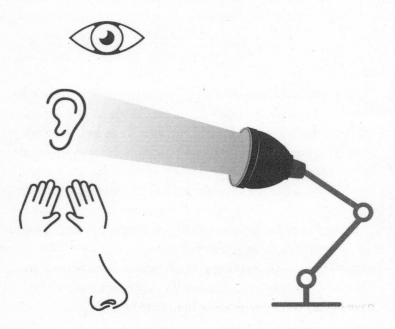

Confidence grows from knowledge

Knowledge is definitely power; fear and stress often melt away once you have an understanding of what is happening to your body and why. Have you ever sat down and talked to someone about your changing physiology at this time of your life? It almost certainly wasn't part of your sex education classes, and is unlikely to have come up in a discussion at the pub. Most women have never sat down and had a lesson on their hormones, and certainly have not been taught in a formal way about the changes that can happen during the years leading up to menopause. It has recently been announced that teaching on menopause will become part of the national curriculum and there are movements within trade unions and the corporate sector to regard experiences of menopause in the workplace as something to be supported. So, there is hope!

Wider acceptance means that sharing experiences becomes less of a taboo. Shared experiences are a vital part of reducing fear and increasing confidence in knowing that you can, and will, manage to survive and even thrive during this stage of your life. When I started having some quite intense experiences, I actively started quizzing women who had been through menopause. Talking to women that had, or were going through, a very positive and empowering experience was very different from listening to those who came to see me because they were having difficulties. This insight into how differently women experienced menopause gave me a unique overview.

Like an easy birth, how many women openly discuss when they have had an easy time of it? If their friends are having a difficult time, it feels lacking in empathy to say, 'mine was fine'. But we really do need to hear inspiring stories of women who have had a positive experience of menopause.

If someone says to me 'it was fine', I want to know more and I'm not afraid to ask women more about their experience if it comes up in conversation, or even when it doesn't. Knowing others have been through that experience, and not only survived, but also thrived can really change your perspective.

I invite you to imagine this transitional time as a gear change in a car. In a car that isn't being well maintained, the gears might stick and be harder to change, whereas in a well-maintained car the gear switch can be a lot smoother. Imagine how much easier your journey will be when you understand the mechanisms and learn how to maintain them optimally.

By understanding these aspects of menopause and learning more of what your body can do, and is doing, you will start to feel your fear decrease and your confidence increase. Your belief in your ability to navigate the ups and downs of perimenopause will become stronger, making you more resilient.

EXERCISE 24: MAKING IT A POSITIVE PAUSE

Allow yourself five to ten minutes to consider the aspects of menopause that are positive to you. I'm not going to suggest any as I want them to come from within you.

_____

_____

_____

If you can't think of any now, that's okay; as you read this book, other positive aspects may come into your mind as you begin to turn your attention to new possibilities.

'I fearlessly embrace the changes
that are happening in my life.'

The power of socialisation

There is an important aspect of our society called 'socialisation' – broadly defined, it's the process of transferring norms, values, beliefs and behaviours to future members of a particular group in society. You may have understood it in the past in relation to children and how they learn to socialise, but socialisation can apply to many groups in society – and it also applies to the years leading up to menopause and beyond.

With effective socialisation, we learn from the groups that have already been through that experience – just as children learn from older peers or parents. Women like you, moving through a midlife transition, will look to the group before them to understand their experience and adapt. If you are fortunate to have a mother, other women in your family, or friends to talk to, have you spoken to them about their experiences?

Bringing groups of women together to discuss their experiences of menopause in a nurturing and supportive way enables those that have been through the transition to nurture others through it.

'It's the most wonderful f··king thing in the world . . . no
longer a slave, no longer a machine with parts. You're just
a person, in business . . . it is horrendous, but then it's
magnificent. Something to look forward to.'

Belinda in *Fleabag*

Transition and uncertainty

During a life transition it's normal to feel some level of fear and excitement, or both! For example, moving to a new house, starting a new job or getting married signify a shift in your world and all have an element of the unexpected woven into them. Yet with all of those intentional transitions you are choosing to make a commitment and change. You have invested in your future emotionally or financially. You play it safe or take a risk – but you have made a choice. Even when you make a choice out of love, desire, trust or from a place of hope, it is normal to feel apprehensive. This is how change is.

Then there are the transitions that you have no choice over, more existential transitions that are part of being human. The shifts and changes marked by time are unavoidable, powerful and meaningful. Sometimes you may get a sense of the change but feel 'out of sorts' as if things aren't quite right, or you're not yourself. Some women say, 'It feels as if I have no control over my own body'.

The good news is that you do still have some control – while you can't choose to stop menopause, you can choose how you respond to it.

Some people are not aware of these shifts psychologically, and others are very engaged and proactive in experiencing that change – perhaps excited about the growth that a transitional stage offers. It's no coincidence that you are reading these words right now – usually people find their way to my books because they sense the shifts they are experiencing and want to be more connected to the changes that are happening.

Stress, fear and your body

Stress can have a profound impact on your experience. Many aspects of perimenopause such as anxiety, hot flushes, mood changes, even changes in your bone density, can be impacted by stress, in particular social stress.

To understand why managing stress, worry and fear is so important in relation to perimenopause, it helps to understand how your body responds to stress.

Meet your stress hormones: adrenaline (epinephrine), noradrenaline (nor-epinephrine) and cortisol. This little bunch of hormones is designed to regulate your responses to danger, via your sympathetic nervous system (your stress system or hot head) and your parasympathetic nervous system (your soothing system or cool head). I'm also going to introduce you to something called GABA, an amino acid also known as a neurotransmitter. GABA has a really important role and learning how to take care of and nurture it will help you to reduce stress, thereby reducing the intensity of some menopausal experiences.

GABA's role in the body is to regulate the activity of neurons in the brain and central nervous system, which in turn has a broad range of effects, including increased relaxation, reduced stress, a more calm, balanced mood, alleviation of physical discomfort and a boost to sleep. Sounds good doesn't it?

GABA is your friend but it faces a few challenges during perimenopause, so it's up to you to get to know what those challenges are and learn how you can support them. The challenges occur because of progesterone. Progesterone is mostly produced by your adrenal glands, which are located near your kidneys and are the same part of your body that produces adrenaline, noradrenaline and cortisol, the stress hormones. These travel through your blood to your brain and are able to cross what is known as the blood–brain barrier.

In perimenopause, even when you are calm and relaxed, progesterone will drop, and as it drops it impacts on GABA. This may trigger anxiety, depression, mood changes and sleep issues. If this happens it's not uncommon to feel more anxious in certain situations, to feel stressed with not enough sleep, or to be reactive to certain situations. By this I mean shouting at your family, being short with colleagues or friends, and then feeling terrible about an overreaction a few minutes later. If your life is busy, and you are balancing many things, it may feel very overwhelming, and this stress response can be heightened. When the stress response is heightened the body needs adrenaline and noradrenaline to help us stay alert and get out of danger. It also needs cortisol.

Where are all these stress hormones produced? You've guessed it, in the adrenals. If your body needs more cortisol, the adrenal glands have to get it from somewhere. And this is where it gets problematic as already low progesterone stores are converted to cortisol. If you are in a persistent state of stress or heightened anxiety, it can put pressure on your adrenal glands, increase cortisol and reduce progesterone. This in turn impacts on GABA, which doesn't receive the progesterone it needs to keep you happy, calm and relaxed.

Fight, flight and freeze – and fawn

Human beings are mammals; you are a mammal. Never forget that you are part of an amazing species that has survived and evolved over thousands of years. To stay safe and survive, humans need a top-notch alert system – a stress system. To survive you need to be able to adapt quickly to situations that pose danger. If in danger, any mammal, including you, has a survival response that kicks in so you can fight or run away, or freeze.

This is where your amygdala makes its grand entrance. Imagine this part of your brain as a small almond shape deep in the oldest part of your brain. Your amygdala is attuned to fear; it's your protector. It's the part that activates the stress system if it senses danger.

We instinctively fear certain things such as snakes, and we can feel anxious when we're about to cross a busy road; this is perfectly normal and is our amygdala telling us to take care. However, the amygdala has become more active than it should be as our lives have become busier and more complicated and we have become overwhelmed and stressed by day-to-day life. Because of this, facing a huge pile of paperwork or someone asking things of you when you feel exhausted can be as threatening as a tiger!

Stress can also be mistaken for anger – for example, in fight or flight response you might snap at your loved ones. Your body is giving you an early warning sign, so this is the time to start thinking about what you need and prioritise self-care.

Learning to recognise when your stress system is triggered will help you to learn when to activate your soothing system. Turning down stress and recognising where there is overwhelm in your life can help you support your whole body and mind during your menopause transition. It may mean making some tough decisions, but isn't the priority a life that you don't want to run away from, but one where you can feel happy, secure, relaxed and safe?

A simple daily meditation can actually shrink the amygdala in size, while your responsive pre-frontal cortex, the executive, regulatory part of your brain, becomes stronger. This builds resilience.

When you are feeling stressed or under pressure the prospect of finding time for meditation may feel challenging, but the more you do it the less challenging it becomes and the more you feel the benefit in your daily life.

'You should sit in meditation for 20 minutes every day – unless you're too busy; then you should sit for an hour.'

Old Zen proverb

Slightly different from all of this is the fawn response. This is a fourth aspect of the survival response that we see in our society as people become afraid to voice their opinion or speak up. If you are always people-pleasing, scared to say what you really think, or constantly flattering others to avoid conflict, this may be your fawn stress response. A fawn response means that you say 'yes' a lot and find it hard to say 'no'. It's one that I see shifting in perimenopause and definitely post-menopause, so start noticing this pattern and become a 'no person', someone who is able to stand up for their convictions and who isn't afraid of conflict.

'What works to address all these emotions is, I've found, not putting up with bullshit from others, saying it how it is, being authentic and not making excuses for yourself. As well as looking after your physical body with exercise, good food, complementary therapies and supplements. Alongside this I've also noticed a change in myself as I become more reflective, grounded in my experiences and less reactive.'

Laura

Breaking the cycle of stress

Now that you know that stress without an outlet can build up and affect you physically, it's time for you to learn how you can let go of stress and disrupt that cycle in the moment. Self-hypnosis is a great tool for rapid changes in the moment, but the power is in being able to create sustainable and long-lasting habits that can make a difference each and every day. If you were given a course of medicine for 14 days and only took it on the days you remembered, it wouldn't be as effective as it's meant to be would it?

EXERCISE 25: NAME IT TO TAME IT

This little exercise will help you to manage difficult feelings and give you some simple ways to weave this into your life. If difficult feelings are coming up, such as conflict, anger or frustration, notice them and then let the emotional charge go.

- Sit somewhere on a chair with your feet on the ground and take a few deep breaths – use the grounding exercise on page 58 if you need to.
- If your mind wanders, come back to your breath.
- Breathe in and breathe out.
- Notice how you are feeling; perhaps you are restless, calm, uncomfortable, comfortable.
- Name the feelings as they arise – even an itch or an ache can be named and noticed.
- As you accept and name those feelings just as they are in that moment, they start to lose their emotional charge.

As you become more used to this, you'll feel calmer and more in control in moments when you previously felt stressed and anxious. The more you do this, the stronger this muscle becomes and the more rested and calmer your amygdala is.

EXERCISE 26: LETTING GO OF STRESS

See page 9 for download link.

A hypnosis visualisation can help you to relax and unconsciously let go of anything that is causing you stress and anxiety. This is a great exercise to do at the end of the day. If you are struggling to fit any downtime in, you can listen to it in bed before you go to sleep. The benefit of this is that you will likely fall into a deep restful sleep afterwards.

Tip: Be creative. Each time you have a bath imagine that when you pull the plug you are getting rid of accumulated stress, or that when you vacuum your home that every bit of dust or crumb on the floor is stress from your day. Vacuuming it up clears your home and your mind of stress.

EXERCISE 27: MAKING IT SUSTAINABLE

Reducing stress is not just about a meditation practice or using hypnosis tools, it's also about self-care. This exercise is about creating a daily, weekly and monthly habit of looking after yourself by doing things that bring you pleasure; little acts of self-kindness. You can add these to your self-care prescription on page 170.

Daily: What small acts of calm could you do daily? Think of moments that give you time to focus on your well-being. It may be sitting down for a quiet cup of tea, going for a walk, having a conversation with a friend, drawing, listening to a podcast or an audiobook.

1. _____

2. _____

3. _____

Weekly: There may be some things that you can only really do once a week. It may be catching up with a friend, going for a long run. These little acts of self-care may take a little longer. Write down three things that take a little longer, but lift you up.

1. _____

2. _____

3. _____

Monthly: Sometimes we need to treat ourselves to something special. How often do you do this? Consider booking a day off work so you can have a long weekend or a night away, going to the theatre or a concert, or even planning a weekend with nothing booked in at all! It can really help to get something in the diary so that this time is ring-fenced.

1. _____

2. _____

3. _____

Summary

Learn to recognise the signs of stress building up, and how to let go of fear or anxiety on a daily basis. Remember letting go of everyday worries stops them building up and becoming overwhelming. Find ways of prioritising your well-being, even if it means ensuring it's a regular date in the diary. Set yourself a reminder! Start to make self-care a normal part of your daily life. And . . . put boundaries in place; if your gut is saying no, say 'no'. Accept that some days you can't do everything that others expect of you, but you can take care of yourself.

6

Belief and Expectation

Hokusai says look carefully.
He says pay attention, notice.
He says keep looking, stay curious.
He says there is no end to seeing
He says look forward to getting old.
He says keep changing, you just get more who you
really are.

Roger Keyes, from the poem 'Hokusai Says'

What do you believe to be true about menopause? What stories have you heard that have shaped your view of it? In the last chapter you learned how your thoughts and feelings can influence physical experiences in your body, so even though 'it's all in your mind', it doesn't lessen what you are experiencing.

Past experiences often shape future ones, but they don't have to. Your beliefs about menopause can define whether you have a negative or positive experience of it.

The subtitle of this book is 'Hypnosis and Mindfulness Tools for a Calm and Confident Menopause'. When you chose to buy it, part of you believed that this was possible or that it was something you would like to experience. The choice you made is an important one as it tells me that you have already started to believe that you can have a calm and confident menopause.

Let's take a look at how those beliefs are formed and why they matter.

Learning your menopause bias

One of the most important factors in belief and experience is unconscious bias, something that is part of being human. There is so much information in the world that your brain would become overwhelmed if you tried to process it all. Instead, you will have defined beliefs and values that help you navigate the world around you more easily. These will have shaped your friendship groups, your work, your hobbies and your attitudes to politics and religion.

Confirmation bias is your brain's way of ensuring that the world around you makes sense. It's as if your brain were playing a giant game of snap with what you believe internally and things that you experience externally in the world around you. Anything that doesn't fit is filtered out before you even become aware of it.

Importantly, this mostly happens automatically, so to change an attitude or behaviour you have to change your values and beliefs at an unconscious level.

Imagine that you have an infinite experience library in your mind that stores all the things you have been told, seen, read, heard or even experienced around menopause. They are all squirrelled away in a section called 'menopause'. When you are young it may be quite empty, but as you grow older it begins to fill up with stories from friends or family and also media, cultural references and education. Now this is where it gets interesting – your brain knows that you are nearing midlife and knows about menopause, so it begins to search for more information that aligns it with that knowledge. You will start to filter out stories and messages related to different stages in your life, such as motherhood, and start to filter in messages about midlife. You may notice more coverage on radio or television shows, books, podcasts, or even articles in magazines and newspapers about menopause – it's likely that it is the same amount as it's always been; it will just seem as if it's more because you are more tuned into it.

This reference system in your brain is outside of your conscious awareness, which is why your environment can have such an impact on your experience. To change your belief and shift your bias you need to bring it into your conscious awareness.

Where focus goes energy flows

Here are two examples of how expectation can shape your experience of menopause.

Ivy believes that she doesn't want to experience menopause, not least because her best friend has told her 'it's the worst'. She's told Ivy how her experiences are impacting on her relationships, wearing her down, how depressed she is feeling; how she feels redundant now that her children have gone to university. She uses language, like 'no end in sight', and describes feeling 'washed up' and 'invisible'. As Ivy listens to her friend, she begins to wonder if when she was feeling warm last week it was a hot flush, and starts to think, 'Yes, that was an unpleasant feeling.' Her belief starts to form, and her attention starts to focus on what she is experiencing physically. She becomes tired and thinks 'Is this it? Is my sleep disturbed?' As she focuses more on physical changes, perhaps starting to feel anxious, she may begin to notice the same

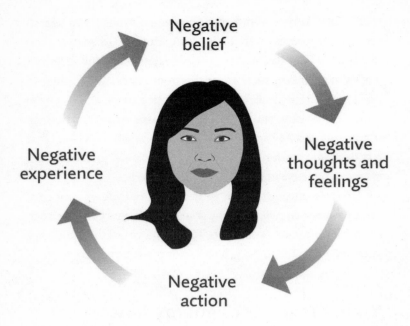

Negative
belief

Negative
thoughts and
feelings

Negative
action

Negative
experience

experiences as her friend, and the impact of them on her relationships and her feelings and experience begin to change as well.

Joy is looking forward to this life stage. She's surrounded by a mix of people, but most of her friends are positive about the changes that are happening to them. Joy's children are off to university and she sees this as an opportunity to start a new hobby and go on more holidays – now they have left the nest, it's time for her to spread her wings. She goes walking with a group of friends twice a week, and they talk about all their experiences. She notices the changes that are happening in her body, but she doesn't regard them as something to be afraid or anxious about – rather something to be aware of. She listens to what her body is telling her, is forgiving towards herself for her sometimes quick temper, and when she is tired she chooses to rest.

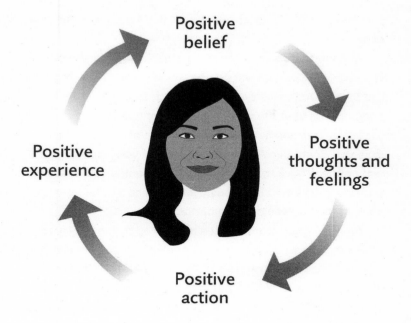

Positive
belief

Positive
experience

Positive
thoughts and
feelings

Positive
action

Happily, you can decide to be Joy not Ivy! By taking charge of the information that you receive, you can begin to change it. You can do this by:

1. Changing your internal narrative
2. Changing external messages
3. Actively engaging with different groups of people
4. Changing your language

Changing your internal narrative

Thoughts and feelings play a leading role in the theatre of your menopause transition; they can be the hero or the villain. As you go through perimenopause and beyond, your inner narrator is part of the script-writing team; its voice matters and can make all the difference to what you feel, and what you experience.

That internal voice can be noisy and chatty, it can be reflective and quiet, or it can be compassionate and loving. Most of the time though this part of the mind is critical. Your inner critic reflects your inner bias around menopause and is often fuelled by fear and anxiety. It can cast doubt on your abilities, stop you doing things that are outside of your comfort zone and hold you back from fulfilling your potential. It often stops you taking risks, which can be positive, but also stifles your creativity and shuts the door on opportunity.

Your inner narrator has been influenced by messages from others in the past that you aren't good enough, that you've got it wrong, that everyone does 'it' so much better, or that everything you have achieved has been luck. How often do you stand in front of the mirror and love your body along with all the changes that are happening? Do you see that you are a wise, skilled multitasker? Do you stop at the end of the day and hear your inner voice say, 'You did a great job today'?

When you hear a negative voice in your head, think, 'Where have I heard that before?', 'Who has said that to me?' It may be something a teacher, a parent, someone at school, even a boss or a partner has said to you – those messages stick. Your inner narrator echoes those messages as they are learned patterns, but they can also be unlearned.

EXERCISE 28: WORKING WITH YOUR INNER CRITIC

Your inner critic needs to feel safe and loved, and to know that you are okay. Get to know it and befriend it. You are on the same team. Recognising the negative patterns and letting them go means that you can work together to create new healthy and supportive patterns.

You can fill in the lines below or do this exercise in your journal if you prefer.

Week one: Listen to your inner narrator for a week and write down what it is saying to you. Is there a similar pattern?

_____

_____

_____

_____

Make a pact with your inner narrator to let the old pattern go. Imagine that you are working together, creating a shared goal. You can even imagine it as a contract that you both choose to sign.

Week two: In the second week, every time a negative message comes up, notice it, stop it and change it into a positive message. Going forward be alert to that 'little voice inside your head'. Whenever it is negative, remind it of your pact and change the narrative. Write down the positive statements that emerge from this inner dialogue.

_____

_____

_____

'I look at my achievements with loving awareness.'

EXERCISE 29: GROWTH AFFIRMATIONS

On page 38 I introduced affirmations. When it comes to changing beliefs, they are a great tool to help you get into a positive state of mind. This exercise is about growth affirmations – those that help you grow internally, not just change a belief. I've given you some examples of growth affirmations, opposite, but the best ones are those you write yourself because they are congruent. This means they are more in tune with your expectations, so they will be easier to stick to.

Rule one is that an affirmation should always be affirmative! If I were to say to you, 'Whatever you do, don't turn around'. What do you want to do? Turn around of course! When you write an affirmation and say, 'I don't want to feel tired', all your brain will hear is 'feel tired'. In fact, you may already be feeling tired as your attention goes to tiredness. Instead, write an affirmation that reads, 'When I take a deep breath in, I am energised'. The message your brain hears is 'I am energised'.

The more you practise affirmations, the more they become part of your thinking. Clients often come back to me reciting their affirmations mid-sentence without realising. This shows me they have become an intrinsic part of their belief system and a physical experience.

Here are a few to start you off:

- The unknown is bringing me opportunities to grow.
- I am comfortable with change.
- I am open to positive experiences of peri/menopause.
- Every experience I have reminds me of my growing power.
- I am the person I always was, and more.
- I love the wise woman I am growing into.

Now add your own . . .

_____

_____

_____

_____

There are more affirmations scattered throughout the book – either use them as they are or adapt them. If you have a specific aspect of perimenopause you are finding challenging, write a positive affirmation to counterbalance the negative feeling, thought or experience. For example, if you find hot flushes stressful and uncomfortable, the affirmation might be 'Each time I have a hot flush I am aware of my wisdom rising/power surging.'

Taking ownership of your affirmations is important as they become even more powerful when they come from you. Would they make a positive impact if you record and listen to them instead of, or as well as, writing them down? Think about which format would work best for you.

🎧 There are also recorded affirmation tracks that you can download at www.penguin.co.uk/mindfulmenopause.

Changing your external narrative

Once you have thought about the messages you receive internally about menopause, start to think about the external messages. By that I mean things that people say to you or that you read in newspapers or magazines and books. There are prevalent ideas about menopause in our culture that you will have absorbed both consciously and unconsciously. This work is not about hypnotising you into a positive experience; it's about de-hypnotising you of negative messages you have been receiving all your life.

You may have seen the British mentalist Derren Brown make use of this function of our brain regularly to plant suggestion in staged performances. It's called perception without awareness. What it means is that there are things outside your immediate attention that can affect your beliefs and behaviour? For example, when Derren Brown wants someone to think of the number 3, he may have a picture of 3 vases on the wall, a room with the door number 3 or 33, or put 3 people next to the person he is influencing. When he says give me a number between 1 and 10, the person is very likely to choose 3.

When it comes to menopause, the odds don't seem to be stacked in our favour as the cultural messages around it are largely negative. Even 'positive' humour by women around menopause is disparaging. However, you can still do a lot to change the external messages you receive, which can affect your experience.

EXERCISE 30: WHAT MESSAGES ARE YOU HEARING?

First, identify where you hear messages that make you feel despondent, disempowered and anxious about menopause. Consider the three most frequent sources of these messages – it may be friends, social media, medical staff, family.

1. _____

2. _____

3. _____

Now think about how you can change the messages you are receiving. It may be changing the channels you subscribe to, befriending other women that are very positive about this life stage, or reading books that have a gentle, empowering and positive outlook of menopause.

Sometimes you can't avoid certain people or groups and you know that they are going to be talking negatively about midlife. It might be a group of friends, work colleagues or family. If you aren't able to remove the information you are receiving, you can learn how to change it. What if you could change the conversation, change the story from the first comment?

The next tool is a very useful one for conversations that make you feel uncomfortable or drain you because they feel inconsistent with the helpful, kind, inspiring or reassuring messages you want to hear about menopause.

EXERCISE 31: YOUR MENOPAUSE FILTER

This is a very simple self-hypnosis tool. Imagine that there is a cloud between you and the other person who is speaking; it's a bit like a filter – any words or phrases that pass through the filter and are incongruent with the experience you want to shape become jumbled and meaningless, perhaps even disappearing. Your mind finds it easy to take control of your experience, and it becomes an important reminder of your power in this situation to manage the stories that cross your path.

Practise this exercise first, somewhere that you feel calm and comfortable. It works on the basis that you can control what you choose to hear and how you receive that information. You can choose to let it go. Once you have practised it, you can do it without even having to close your eyes, or anyone else noticing.

- Take a deep breath in and close your eyes.
- Imagine a mist with an inbuilt filter. It can be white, or you can give it a colour that represents change or positivity to you.
- As that person/group is talking, imagine all the words going through the filter.
- As they do, the words soften and lose their power.
- Notice how the energy of the words change.
- Allow your mind to delete or get rid of those unhelpful words, phrases or stories in a way that's right for you – you can be as creative as you like!

Close your eyes now and imagine a situation in which this would be helpful. As always be playful with these kinds of visualisations, and work with your imagination.

Washing it all off

At the end of the day, if you have a shower you can imagine washing any negative energy off. If you are someone who feels connected with smell, use a soap with a scent that you associate with attributes such as fortitude, clarity, wisdom, feeling beautiful or calm. As you wash, imagine washing off all the negative energy you may have come into contact with that day and enjoy watching it disappear down the plughole.

Changing it up!

Sometimes changing things up and introducing something new and different into your life will be easier. First think about what you can change.

Can you join clubs or find a new hobby or activity, with people that have a very positive outlook? This is something I really encourage, and have seen many people benefit from – it's stimulating, energising and sociable. I have known clients take up tennis in their 60s. Doing something that makes you feel fit and healthy, both physically and cognitively, can change your embodied beliefs.

Join a positive menopause group online or follow some accounts that empower and lift you up. There are plenty of great accounts to follow – you'll find some suggestions on page 311 to get you started. Perhaps even start your own account of your positive journey to inspire other women!

Make sure that the balance of information you are receiving is weighted towards feeling positive and empowered by this life transition. Your infinite experience library (see page 126) needs to be filled up with messaging and experiences that you can aspire to and feel good about. When you do this, you will notice more and more positive messages as your filter changes to align itself with your new positive belief.

Your brain is incredible – it does all this without you even realising. After a few weeks of changing beliefs by using these tools, it's not uncommon to hear my clients say something like, 'I feel so much better, it must be because the sun is shining today.' Nothing to do with the hypnotherapy, of course!

The language of menopause

The final, but one of the most important, pieces of the belief jigsaw is how you talk about menopause. The words you use hold power and the brain communicates often in a surprisingly literal way. Here's one example of this:

One of my client's was experiencing insomnia as part of her menopausal experience. She just couldn't sleep. She was on HRT and had been taking sleeping tablets to no avail. We had a chat, and she told me about a fire that had broken out at her home the year before. The firemen were quick to arrive and put the fire out; the house was quickly made safe. She said the firemen were lovely and reassuring, and as they turned to leave one of them said to her, 'You are lucky you were awake as otherwise you would have died.'

Immediately I knew that the insomnia was not related to menopause. Her brain listened to the fireman and, in a state of disruption and high arousal, all it heard was, 'If you had been asleep, you would have died.' I simply reflected that back to her followed by doing some quick hypnosis to help her let it go. She was soon sleeping again.

Other things I hear in my clinic a lot are 'I am menopausal', 'I have night sweats all the time', 'I am anxious all the time.' Think about the belief and expectation that sits behind these phrases.

- You are not menopausal – you are having some experiences that may be part of perimenopause.
- You are not having night sweats all the time – you may be having some sweats during some nights.
- You are not anxious all the time – you have moments when you experience anxiety more than others.

Often the first, and easiest step to changing your experience is changing your language around it. Make your experience a temporary state that you can learn to accept and let go of as you learn to eliminate it from your life completely.

EXERCISE 32: DON'T PARAPHRASE, POWERPHRASE

It's not uncommon for people to use phrases that they often hear and these are likely to reflect the cultural attitude to their experience. A friend recently came back from the doctor and said to me, 'I've been diagnosed with menopause.' These words speak volumes, as they suggest menopause is a disease or an illness, something to be treated.

Set yourself a task for a few days and notice if you come out with any disempowering phrases or words around midlife or menopause. If you do, think about how you could rephrase them and write them down here.

_____

_____

_____

Tip: You could also write the words and phrases on some sticky notes and place them somewhere that you will see them often.

Words hold meaning and meaning is your connection to expectation and experience.

Summary

Unconscious beliefs are deeply connected to your experience. Learning how to recognise deep-seated beliefs and wanting to change them is a powerful step to reshaping this time of your life. Remember that everyone has their own story based on their values and their experiences. Only you can change your personal value system; only you can change your story. Create a set of positive beliefs that you can live by. Write them down in your journal so you can keep coming back to them.

7

Who Am I Becoming?

You had the power all along my dear.

Glinda, the Good Witch in *The Wizard of Oz* by L. Frank Baum

Although this chapter is in the middle of the book, it's the last one I wrote. For this is where your transition rests, in the essence of who you are in this very moment. We very rarely show our true selves to the world – very few people really know who we truly are. During the years leading up to menopause, you sometimes may not even know yourself.

As is true of many transitions, when you descend into these uncharted waters you will rediscover parts of yourself that you haven't see for a while and parts that you never knew existed. When you emerge again you will reintegrate – stronger, wiser and connected with your deep power.

Imagine it like a veil being lifted; you may suddenly get the sense that your needs are important, and start to understand how much time and energy you have invested in other people's lives. This may have been necessary at some points of your life, tipping the balance of care more frequently towards others than to yourself.

'I'm experiencing something akin to the feeling you may get when you're surrounded by a fog for many years and then the fog begins to lift slowly like a veil, like I am slowly but surely being unveiled . . . I'm feeling a sense of relief and space. My vision is farsighted now, I am relaxed and anxious all at the same time as I embark upon my journey.'

Charmaine

This 'seeing' is experienced by people in many different ways. Some see the cracks that they unconsciously papered over in their lives; some feel a sense of expansion and opportunity; some feel a need to escape. Nearly everyone I speak to talks of anger – this can be expressed in many different ways, and is often dismissed as, 'Oh it's just menopause.' If you are feeling this way, don't be fobbed off with these sorts of comments. There is much more beneath the surface fuelling this, and I'm going to give a brief insight into why we might be so angry!

Throughout history, women's mental health has been a way to subjugate and control then, both at home and in society. In hypnosis history, some of the earliest applications of hypnosis, or mesmerism as it was known, dealt with 'women's hysteria'. 'Symptoms' that led to a diagnosis of hysteria were anxiety, insomnia, loss of sexual appetite and, as one medical book suggested, 'a tendency to cause trouble for others'. Recognise any of those?

Rather than being an equal partner, women were expected to be demure and obsequious. Most people can finish the sentence,' A woman's place is . . . '. *The Good Wife Guide*, published in 1955, has a list of requirements such as, 'Arrange his pillow and offer to take off his shoes. Speak in a low, soft, soothing and pleasant voice. Allow him to relax and unwind'. With the final bullet point being, 'A good wife always knows her place'.

In Switzerland women only got the vote in the 1971. In the mid-1980s my newly divorced mother was told by her bank that she needed her husband with her to sign the mortgage, even though it was based on her own earnings and the house was bought independently.

'Difficult women' made life challenging for others. Even today women are sedated with self-administered tranquillisers and still oppressed depending on where in the world they live. We have been conditioned into experiencing our feelings selectively – caring and nurturing are fine, but anger and frustration are not. Tears are unacceptable, emotion is a weakness. Openness, assertiveness and outspoken behaviour are unwomanly characteristics. Moodiness and 'dysfunction' are seen as a sign of ill health.

> 'I'm not moody, I'm just not putting up with the sh*t I've always put up with.'
>
> Jenny

This is the thinking upon which our culture has grown, and it still persists both consciously and unconsciously in the attitudes of those around us. Even if you have felt that you were a feminist, as you go through perimenopause you may feel for the first time just how limited you have been by the thinking of those around you. It may go as far back as teachers, parents, partners or, more recently, at work.

Where there are women there is power. And where there is power there is fear. Fear can be felt by those whose stability is threatened by those of us who are powerful, but there is also fear of our own power. Marianne Williamson summed this up perfectly when she wrote, 'Our deepest fear is not that we are inadequate. Our deepest fear is that we are powerful beyond measure.'

Having been fortunate to attend many women in moments of true power and strength – such as during birth or in midlife groups – I have seen this intense power, but I have also witnessed discomfort from others when witnessing the expression of this incredible energy. More than once, I have seen women in a place of power offered medication, to quieten down, to fix what wasn't broken. In truth, when you are pushed as far as you think you can go, and then take that one step further you become stronger. That is where growth happens.

Your body and your mind have something similar to a fuel tank warning system. When we are working hard at something, it gives you a warning at around 70 per cent. That's the 'I can't do this anymore' feeling, but you've actually got 30 per cent left in the tank! It's during the hero's journey, your transition, that you learn what your real capacity is.

This time can be one of challenge and upheaval as you arrive at a place where you may no longer want to live as the world expects you to live.

🎧 EXERCISE 33: RECLAIMING YOUR POWER

Over the years your power is diminished by others around you. Whenever you feel shamed, belittled, dismissed, rejected, ignored, threatened or bullied, your light may be dimmed. Now it's time to reclaim your power, to let your light shine, and to give voice to the wisdom you have.

The audio download that accompanies this exercise (see page 9) will call your power back from anyone in the past

WHO AM I BECOMING?

that is still holding on to it. As you listen to the audio, you will feel your power returning and growing. You'll feel grounded and connected to your inner wisdom. You can listen to it whenever you feel you need to.

Grief, loss and letting go

The time around menopause can be a time of grief and loss, and of letting go. You may identify yourself as a mother, but your children may be growing up and leaving home. Your 'empty nest' is a reminder of that loss and with it comes the feeling of 'What do I do now and who am I now?' or a resigned 'I'm not needed anymore.' Most of my friends have children who return and often move in again – changing times and circumstance make this stage more unpredictable than it's ever been.

'I've probably been in the perimenopause for about ten years. Most of the symptoms have been mild – sweating at night being the most distinct. The changes in my life however are profound. After 20 years of centring my life around my family and children, the shift away from this as my daughters grow up and leave home is huge. I don't particularly feel a loss of my fertility, but I feel a loss of my role as mother – moving to the sidelines of their lives as partners, friends and peers loom larger and become more important. I also notice a change in myself as I become more reflective, grounded in my experiences and less reactive. However, I also feel rage – against all the injustices in the world, and impatience with those that minimise or dismiss this.'

Laura

You may have wanted children, but menopause may be a sign that this is no longer an option for you. Whether you have had children, or haven't, the end of your periods can embody feelings of loss. You may mourn the ending of it or you may celebrate that you no longer have to tackle PMS, pain and heavy periods if these have been a problem for you.

Infertility grief by Julianne Boutaleb, Clinical Psychologist

For many women the menopause signals the end of their fertility. Even for those who have had the family they desired, it can be unsettling to notice the physical changes menopause brings. While some gratefully say goodbye to their period and the pain and inconvenience it possibly represents, others mourn the now lost opportunity to create or expand their family.

Coming into the menopause when you have a history of infertility or pregnancy loss can be especially difficult. In fact, recent research shows that women who have experienced infertility problems report higher levels of menopausal symptoms and more psychological difficulty with the transition. Physical symptoms such as menstrual flooding and vaginal dryness may trigger you back to experiences of pregnancy loss and sexual difficulties you had when trying to conceive. Witnessing your children have difficulties with menstruation or pregnancy may also remind you of your own unresolved losses. If you have not become a mother when you wanted to be, you may unexpectedly find yourself experiencing complex grief or low mood.

If you experienced any of these issues you may find it helpful to understand that infertility grief is a very common experience in menopause and develop a more compassionate approach to your body, honouring it for how it has served you and what it has been through.

- Discover a hobby that lets you experience your body in new ways, such as yoga, walking, dance.
- Find ways of nourishing your body, such as massage and a healthy diet.
- Develop rituals to commemorate any losses you have experienced in your reproductive life.
- Seek therapeutic support to help you with unresolved issues around infertility and pregnancy loss.

While this sudden space in your life may sometimes feel immobilising, it can be liberating. Where there is loss, there may also be renewal. That's the ambiguity of transition. This chapter will help you to connect with your values, your confidence and to hold out a hand to guide you and help you move forward into the next stage of your life with a deep sense of being rooted in your values and intentions.

EXERCISE 34: A TIME FOR LETTING GO

Keep a jar and post-it notes somewhere that is out of sight, but that you can access easily. Every time a worry or concern comes to mind, write it down and put it in the jar. It may be something from your past or something that is bothering you that day. When you feel ready and you have some head space, tackle the jar. Put music on, get comfortable and relax. Take the worries out one by one and decide what you are ready to let go of that day. When you have chosen one or more, light a small candle somewhere safely, and burn the piece of paper. As you do so say something like, 'It mattered to me once, but now I choose to let it go' or simply 'Thank you and goodbye.'

If the worry starts to come back into your mind, be curious about what has triggered it. Write it down again and put it in the jar. Sometimes once is not enough – we can't properly let it go until we have seen it in all its different forms.

Tip: If you feel it needs a proper thank you and goodbye, write a letter to your worry before letting it go.

🎧 Listening to the Letting Go of Stress audio download (see page 9) may help you to let go of things that are troubling and worrying you. I recommend listening to it at the end of the day before you go to sleep.

A space between

All transitions occur in a space where there is a confluence of two stages of your life – past experiences resonate and future opportunities are being born within it. It feels like the birth of a star. The space is alive with the power of these energies; they are sometimes quiet and sometimes discordant. They flow in and out moment by moment; some days the space can feel crowded and overwhelming and other days peaceful. These are your disappointments, your hurts, broken relationships, waistlines that are now a distant memory, roads not taken, and there may be fear and anxiety of what lies ahead. This energy can swarm around you, but it doesn't have to take over the space. Just be in that space and breathe on the days when it feels like this.

While you are letting go of one stage of your life, the other is reaching out to you, but both will always be a part of you. It's a time to rest, reflect, connect and start your next phase of growth. You are a wanderer in this space, not quite sure where you are heading but on a journey of discovery.

As you exist in these moments, you are given an opportunity to look back on what has passed, to honour yourself and to release things that are an unnecessary burden. It is also the space from which you can prepare to fearlessly step into the person you are becoming, even if it makes you feel vulnerable. The tumult of emotions – weepiness, anger, frustration, an abundance of joy – all powerfully rise up to meet you in this space.

It sometimes feels expectant, as if you are waiting for something, but you don't know quite what or when it will happen. Sometimes it's unsettling, sometimes you can feel grounded. Sometimes you may feel powerless and sometimes powerful. Treat these feelings as a guide; they will show you how you can equip yourself for this next life stage. Test different approaches, notice how you respond – this is you building resilience and tapping into your power.

This is where the spiritual transition meets the physical shift – a chance for your mind, heart and soul to have a conversation and agree on the small adjustments that can be made to create balance in your life.

Learning to lean into this space and be present moment by moment allows transformational energy to find its way into your heart. Welcome it lovingly, in a way that is meaningful to you. An opportunity to connect with joy and love in readiness for what lies beyond sits within this space, patiently waiting for you to unfold into it.

And then suddenly you know you have arrived where you needed to be.

> 'I am exactly where I need to be
> right now.'

Retreat and reflection

Being able to retreat and reflect is a consistent theme and many women confess that they feel a slowing down at this stage of their lives. I've used the word 'confess' deliberately, as we are conditioned to think that if we are not always busy doing something, we are somehow being lazy. You know this isn't true, but this is how you can be made to feel. Now is a time to take refuge in yourself, give expression to who you are and to listen to what you need.

Tip: Try to substitute doing with being. If you find yourself keeping busy because you feel unsettled and anxious, learn to stop for just a minute and simply notice and name the feeling. Use the Name It To Tame It exercise on page 121.

If you find that you are unable to sit with your feelings even for a minute and keep wanting to 'do' things to fill that space, consider seeing a therapist (see page 83) to explore why this is.

If you have lived at a fast pace, been passionate about work or keen to give as much as you can, you may notice a change in your attention and focus. If you notice this happening, sit with it. This time is a time of reflection – the powerful energy that you are connecting with demands attention. With that attention you can go deeper into yourself, learning where you need to be to arrive at a place of peace. You may also be drawn to use this as a time to take a sabbatical from work or to travel somewhere remote, or perhaps attend retreats and personal development courses.

Reflection may simply take place at home, perhaps by meditating or reading something that calls to you. It may be a place where you write poetry, journal or listen to music. Creating a physical space in which to retreat and reflect helps to remind you of the importance of spending time in meditative or creative practice. This space can be a room, or just the corner of a room, your bedside table or an area by your bed.

Your box of treasure

Having a box where you keep important items that you associate with your retreat space can help you, even if you have very limited space. Find a box that you are drawn to and decorate it if you want to. Keep your menopause journal, books, poetry, pens, crafting items, crystals, cards, shawl, pictures of people that inspire you, affirmations in it – bring whatever is important to you and connects you to the box. Keep the box somewhere to hand, but private if you prefer, so that you can take something out that might help you in any moment.

Connecting with your values

Whichever stage of life you are at, your values stay fairly constant. Sometimes when life is busy and overwhelming, your values may be submerged. At different times of your life some values may apply more, and you may develop new ones at any point. They can be the roots that tether you in a storm, and they may nurture you with familiarity in those moments when you feel adrift.

As you approach decisions or challenges, you can connect with your values to help ground and direct you in a way that feels authentic. Sometimes you need time to connect with that part of you. If you are faced with a difficult choice, or a challenging situation, be patient. Nothing has to happen now. Take the time you need to get in touch with what feels right for you. If may be self-compassion, integrity, honesty, openness. Use your values to centre yourself and get back to who you are before you make a decision. Everyone else can wait.

Tip: Use your breathing, retreat space or box of treasure to help ground and remind you of what is important to you and to connect with your values.

You can approach daily tasks while connected with your values, or you can tackle longer-term goals and plans in line with your values.

EXERCISE 35: YOUR MENOPAUSE VALUES

This is a condensed list of values. If you want to go more deeply into this exercise, you can print off a complete set of values – you'll find the resource for this at www.penguin. co.uk/mindfulmenopause.

Circle ten values that you most identity with and then reduce that to five; if you absolutely can't reduce it to five, keep those that are really important to you. Write them down or do something creative with them, returning to them whenever you need to gain clarity and connect with yourself.

Passion	Openness	Generosity
Integrity	Power	Vision
Patience	Adventure	Truth
Honesty	Balance	Decisiveness
Self-respect	Responsibility	Curiosity
Enthusiasm	Gentleness	Resilience
Compassion	Cheerfulness	Vulnerability
Strength	Forgiveness	Supportive
Commitment	Determination	Kindness
Awareness	Respect	Purpose
Ambition	Creativity	Grace
Love	Sensitivity	Practicality
Perfection	Calmness	Equality
Add your own . . .		

Ignite your autumn queen and crown your crone

Spring, summer, autumn and winter. As our moods are like the seasons, so are our lives. The time around menopause is the autumn of your life, a time for reflection and hibernation, a time when your wisdom grows as you enter into another cycle of growth. You may find that even the colours you wear take on a different hue and that you start to change your look as you claim your crown. You may find that your connection with the earth grows stronger and you begin to gravitate to out-door activities such as gardening or walking. Or you may feel yourself drawn to spirituality in a way that you haven't before. Your creativity can blossom – it can be an opportunity to explore this part of you.

As FSH (see page 80) rises to levels last experienced just before your periods began, you may feel a sense of childish joy return to your life.

> 'I feel like I did when I was 13, I really do. It's like a light-ness of joy, free of the burdens of the world. I feel as if anything is possible again.'
>
> Elaine

These rising FSH levels can also affect the part of your brain that is responsible for visions, dreams and creativity. Many women talk about having visions, or very realistic dreams, at this time of their lives.

> 'In my mid-40s onwards I had visions mostly in dreams, but they also happened when I was relaxed, and I had a powerful one when I was a passenger in a car. They were colourful and absolutely crystal clear. When I was in meditation, things would sometimes emerge, gradually taking shape, so I experienced answers to my questions. The visions were particularly profound between the ages of 45 and 52, but then stopped being so vivid. Sometimes I still get flashes and I'm in my 70s now.'
>
> Alice

Women of their late 40s into their 50s are also sometimes called maga, the female term for magi – the magician, or high priestess. As you move from this stage into cronehood from around the age of 60 onwards, you become a wise elder. This can be a time for awakening, reinvention, discovery or rediscovery. When you allow time for reflection, you can start to reinvent yourself while still staying true to your values.

You may have heard the word 'crone' or expression 'cronehood', but I'm inviting you to challenge your perception of what a crone is. I suspect that you envision an evil, wizened old woman with warts on her nose and a hairy chin! This is conditioning (well perhaps not the hairy chin) and fear.

We first meet the crone, the witch, in fairy tales – usually *Grimms' Fairy Tales*. These were written by men at a time when women were still being burnt at the stake in Europe and a scold's bridle was used as punishment. This contraption was a metal cage that was put over a woman's head to keep her tongue in place to stop her 'nagging'.

Our perception of crones and witchcraft is steeped in persecution and fear. We need to be reading our children and grandchildren books with luminescent older women, who are caring, nurturing, loving, protecting and wise, so that we all learn from a very early age the nature of womanhood all through the years.

When you dive into the etymology of words associated with older women, they are far more positive than the way in which our culture and conditioning presents them. Hag comes from the word 'hagio', which means holy, witch comes from 'wit', which means wise, and crone comes from 'crown'.

When you shed your conditioning of what you have learned about the years ahead and the power you are growing into, and are able to connect with it confidently, you can start to imagine yourself as the powerful woman you are. Sow the seeds of wisdom that have grown within you.

This is a time for self-expression, creativity and self-care. Turn your attention towards yourself, spend time thinking about things that you want to do. Rediscover a passion for something or awaken a passion for something new. Discuss it with your partner or friends, perhaps finding things that you can do together. It doesn't have to be something you do on your own.

Tip: In your journal list five things that you want to do, or that you are interested in that you haven't had time to do before. Pick one or two to start with and, using your Hypnosis Cloud (see page 49) to get into a state of relaxation, visualise yourself doing each one, step by step. If you have created a menopause vision board (see page 196), you can add them to that as well.

As you free yourself from the expectations of others and shake off the burden of conformity, you can be who you really are. You aren't a different person – you are growing and you are more than have ever been.

'I am the woman I have always been, and even more.'

How do you want to be, and what have you valued and respected in others who have been through this life stage? Is there someone about whom you have thought, 'I want to be like that when I'm that age'. What is it about that person that you value? Do they embody values that you can adopt for this transition and beyond?

EXERCISE 36: AWAKEN YOUR AUTUMN QUEEN

This exercise helps you to imbue your awakening autumn queen with qualities that you want to embody in this stage of your life. It's a simple hypnotic visualisation that helps you connect with someone who has the qualities that you value. It can be someone in your life now or someone who has passed on, or it can be someone famous who you admire and respect.

Find somewhere comfortable to do this exercise and use your Calm Breath (see page 45) and your Hypnosis Cloud (see page 49) to get into a state of comfortable relaxation.

1. When you are relaxed, imagine you are standing in front of the person whose qualities you value.
2. Now just notice that person and how they make you feel. Focus on positive feelings – love, comfort, generosity of heart, purpose, creativity. Refer to the list of values on page 153 if it helps.
3. Give each of those values a colour.
4. Now imagine them moving towards you like colourful sparking waves.
5. Feel those values becoming part of you.
6. Take a really deep breath as they move through every part of your body.
7. Notice them take root in your body.
8. As you breathe in and out, the flow of positive energy moves between you and the other person.
9. Notice the connection between you.
10. Thank the person and say goodbye for now.
11. Open your eyes and take a deep breath.

Each time you want to recall these values, close your eyes and imagine that person. Say their name in your head. If you create a strong association between their name and the value, you will be able to just say their name and feel the connection to that value within you.

Tip: It doesn't have to be just one person. If different people have different qualities that are important to you at this stage in your life and moving forward, you can do this with several people in mind!

Ritual and ceremony

Menopause transition is a rite of passage: as you move through perimenopause, you are moving from one group in society to another. Imagine life as a house, and a rite of passage as moving from one room to another. As you do so, you go through what is known as a liminal stage or a threshold moment.

Rites and ceremonies mark those transitions in our lives – more visible ones are school proms or graduations that are celebratory. Menopause as a rite of passage is not marked or celebrated by our culture in the same way, certainly not in the mainstream.

Croning ceremonies or crowning ceremonies, sometimes also known as a saging ceremonies, do exist though and are becoming more popular. You can create your own with a group of friends or like-minded women or use a trained celebrant to arrange one for you.

If you are on you own or have no one like-minded to join you, take elements of the ceremony and do them yourself when you feel the need. Find a way to translate this ceremony into the power of one.

There are certain rituals that can be part of a ceremony:

- Find a song that represents transition.
- Create a space that feels nurturing.
- Release something that marks fertility into water.
- Have a red thread cut at both ends and ask participants to tie it around their wrist.
- Eat nourishing food.
- Include a ceremonial threshold that you can cross.
- Ask those attending to bring something that represents a milestone in your life.

Tip: You can use elements of a croning ceremony at certain points during the years running up to menopause and beyond. Be guided by your intuition.

Self-care and loving kindness rituals

Rituals are sacred in nature; they connect with your spirit or soul and can be both secular and non-secular. Small daily rituals nourish the connection that is growing with this emerging part of you and are an important part of self-care. Think of doing something small every day that recognises and accepts this in a loving way.

Tip: Every morning when you awaken rest your hand on your heart or just below your collarbone, where it is comfortable and say to yourself, 'Thank you, I love you, I am here for you.'

EXERCISE 37: RITUAL AND REFLECTION

This simple exercise is a ritual to do every night before you go to bed, or if you feel stuck you can use it every time you need to ground yourself.

Start by connecting with your breath and imagining that older, wise and loving person who you know from your past or your present. Maybe it's one of the people from your treasure box. Ask them a question along these lines:

- 'How am I doing?'

- 'How can I be more like you today?'

- 'What's holding me back?'

- 'Why do I feel stuck?'

You can also read a loving kindness meditation, known as a Metta meditation. This meditation can be read out loud either every day, or it can just be a loving way to start the week. As you enter into this new chapter, and you find strength in your wisdom and power, you also step into your role as custodian, wise woman and protector of others. This type of Metta meditation is perfect for menopause:

May I be content
May I be wise
May I be at peace
May I be well

May you be content
May you be wise
May you be at peace
May you be well

May all things be content
May all things be wise
May all things be at peace
May all things be well

The moon and menopause

Some of my clients have found grounding themselves in the energy of their moon cycles a bit 'out there', but often once they have done it, they recognise the power in it. The truth is that with hypnosis I am working with the unconscious, what exists out of your present awareness. We get so used to having periods, that we forget how they anchor us to a cyclical rhythm, which is a type of 'holding'. A therapist or a parent may often talk of a 'holding space' because it's in this space that we feel safe and secure.

Periods hold us in a natural cycle and when they stop, we lose a connection with the holding that cycle offers us. The cycles we are in tether us, our emotions rise and fall within them and the familiarity can be unconsciously soothing, whether we like having periods or not.

As periods start to become further apart, your cycle changes. This is when you can turn to the moon whose waxing and waning is an act of holding.

If you are still getting periods, start to do this anyway as it can be a good habit to get into. If you are following the lunar cycle alongside your periods, carry on with those as you are.

EXERCISE 38: MOON MEDITATION

Tune into the moon to familiarise yourself with her cycle.

New: This is the perfect time to reflect on past goals, and to set new ones. Think about a new project or something that you wish to achieve. It can be something very small. It is the perfect time to implement some self-care in preparation for the energy of the waxing moon. If you exercise a lot, perhaps do something lower energy like going for a long walk.

Waxing Crescent: Your energy is higher, so focus on any plans and projects you may have or visualise their completion. Imagine the energy of your intentions moving out like waves into the world.

First Quarter: Take some physical action towards your goal now. Be flexible and be guided by what comes up as you take action.

Waxing Gibbous: Continue to take steps towards what you want to achieve this month, noticing where adaptations and changes may need to be made and leaning into those.

Full: This is when you are at peak energy, and you'll be able to see the benefits of the work you have done. It's a time to feel gratitude and joy.

Waning Gibbous: You'll still see the returns on the work you've done. Perhaps introduce a gratitude practice (see page 36) into your meditation. 'I am glad that . . .'

Last Quarter: This a time for forgiveness, to let go of any negative thoughts or feelings. It's also a time for rest and reflection.

Your lunar cycle

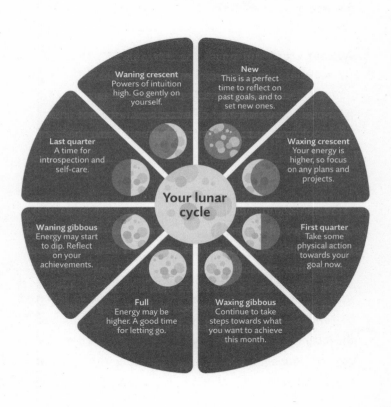

Waning crescent
Powers of intuition high. Go gently on yourself.

New
This is a perfect time to reflect on past goals, and to set new ones.

Last quarter
A time for introspection and self-care.

Waxing crescent
Your energy is higher, so focus on any plans and projects.

Your lunar cycle

Waning gibbous
Energy may start to dip. Reflect on your achievements.

First quarter
Take some physical action towards your goal now.

Full
Energy may be higher. A good time for letting go.

Waxing gibbous
Continue to take steps towards what you want to achieve this month.

Waning Crescent: Reflect on the last month. If you haven't achieved what you set out to do, that's okay. Accept what is beyond your control, let it go and allow yourself to tune into your intuition ready for the next new moon.

Tip: If you are feeling unsettled, then check which moon it is that day and do something that aligns with it. Or just sit with the moon in mind and connect with your breath, grounding yourself in the moon's energy.

Summary

Take this time to go within, and to learn more about yourself. If a thought arises, such as 'I don't even know myself anymore', or you feel lost, without purpose or disconnected, take some time to explore those parts of you. They aren't gone, they are still there. As you expand into this stage of your life, descend into the story of who you are, and what matters to you, rising up stronger and wiser than before. Use the tools in this chapter to help ground you and create a safe haven both within you and around you where you can open yourself up to the journey within. Find ways to express your creativity, ground yourself and to have patience with days that feel full of emotion or that are challenging.

8

Connection and Support

Take my hand. We will walk. We will only walk. We
will enjoy our walk without thinking of arriving
anywhere.

Thich Nhat Hanh

It's not only your beliefs that are important to how you experience the time leading up to menopause; the beliefs of others can also impact on how you feel and how you experience your transition. Connections are important to us as human beings; we are a social species! But you can also manage when you need to without these connections – you can be the cheerleader, the players and the coach for your team of one.

Connections aren't just human connections – there are connections with nature, the world around you and with animals. If you are an animal lover or you have a pet, you already know what a comfort they can be and the unconditional love that they offer.

The connections that I'm going to focus on in this chapter are those with your:

- Self
- Partner
- Children

- Friends and community
- Workplace

The power of oxytocin

Oxytocin is the hormone of love, connection and reproduction – and probably most commonly associated with feeling good. When we have sex, our bodies are awash with oxytocin. When people in the same room as you are experiencing high levels of oxytocin you can too – it's contagious!

Studies have only just started to touch on oxytocin's role in perimenopause, but what we know already is fascinating. Recent studies show many benefits of oxytocin:

- It can improve bone density.
- Oxytocin gel may actually reverse the thinning of the vaginal walls.
- It can reduce cortisol, the stress hormone.

There is even a study that shows frequent hugs, increasing oxytocin levels in women during perimenopause, are linked to lower blood pressure and heart rate.

Oxytocin isn't just the reproductive hormone of birth and sex; it's also important for human beings and social behaviour. Our species needs communities to survive, it's how we have grown. Everyone has roles in society and love literally does make our world go around – it is part of our compassion system. Compassion is an intrinsic part of who you are and plays a vital role in how others make you feel. When you feel supported by the people around you in a loving environment, you produce oxytocin. It thrives best in an environment in which you feel safe, secure and loved.

What's important during perimenopause is to know that oxytocin is not a great friend of adrenaline, and noradrenaline your fight/flight/freeze hormones (see page 118). If your stress levels are high, you produce lower levels of oxytocin, but if your oxytocin is high you reduce the amount of stress hormones in your body – which is fantastic news. When you learn to create opportunities to raise oxytocin during the years leading up to menopause and beyond, you create a loving flow of energy that will have a positive impact on any other experiences you may be having.

During menopause, it seems that as oestrogen drops off so does oxytocin, but the interplay of this is not understood as the research is in its infancy. We do know that oxytocin can still be generated by introducing love and connection into your life. Simply by imagining a loving person nearby, you can experience a spike in oxytocin.

> 'I pay attention to my needs and
> care for myself lovingly.'

EXERCISE 39: THAT LOVING FEELING

Bring someone into your mind that you have felt tremendous love from. It can be anyone from your past, whether that was a fleeting encounter or someone that was in your life for a while. It can be a parent, a friend, a grandparent, a partner. If the person has passed on, the love you received from them will still be very much alive and something you will still be able to draw on – it's a beautiful gift that will keep on giving.

Close your eyes and imagine that person standing or sitting nearby. Notice how they are, perhaps the clothes they are wearing, what they are doing. There may be mannerisms, a smile or a touch, that remind you of the love you felt from them. Allow your heart space to open to that love, notice the feeling of love, how that person made you feel. Allow yourself to sit in this love for a few minutes.

When you open your eyes, write down three words that spring to mind when you feel that love:

1. _____

2. _____

3. _____

These are three things you may need in order to boost your experience of oxytocin. Think about how you can introduce them into your life in other ways.

Try doing this simple exercise on a regular basis. Studies show that it can also increase your compassion and love towards others around you, which then flows back to you.

Be your own cheerleader

Before building a network of connections and a team that you know can help support you on the days you need it most, you have to start with yourself.

I'm guessing that you usually come last on the list of people you need to care for. Self-care is one of those things we all know we should be doing on a daily basis but don't. The phrase 'self-care isn't selfish' is often seen as a meme on social media, but the subtext of this is the belief that caring for yourself is somehow selfish. When did this happen? The truth is that caring for yourself is the foundation of being well enough to care for others. If you are on a plane that is coming down and you have dependants, you always put your own mask on first.

This is all about connecting with your needs – what makes you feel rested, loved, happy, safe, energised or inspired? If you think, 'I haven't got time to care for myself,' then you definitely need to put your oxytocin mask on and do the self-care exercise overleaf.

To find that time you may have to learn the art of the unapologetic 'No', choosing what you give to others in terms of your time, wisely. You may not always be able to say no, especially if you are caring for children or elderly parents, but you don't have to say yes straight away – if you need something in that moment, make sure your immediate needs are met before meeting other people's. If you hear yourself saying, 'Oh I was just about to make a cup of tea . . . ', then make the cup of tea before helping the other person. These are micro-priorities, but they are so important in creating little moments of self-care that make a big difference.

Self-care doesn't need to take a lot of time; it can be five or ten minutes here or there. The next short exercise helps you to focus on what you need. I can't tell you what that is because you are completely unique, so you are going to write your own self-care prescription.

EXERCISE 40: SELF-CARE PRESCRIPTION

Your self-care prescription is a list of things that you know you benefit from. It can be reading 50 pages of a book, having your nails done, meeting up with a friend, crafting, singing, having a relaxing bath. I want you to think of three things that take ten minutes, three things that take 30 minutes and three things that take an hour or longer. Make sure that there are at least two on the list that don't cost anything.

10 minutes or less

1. _____

2. _____

3. _____

30 minutes or less

1. _____

2. _____

3. _____

More than 1 hour

1. _____

2. _____

3. _____

Self-care

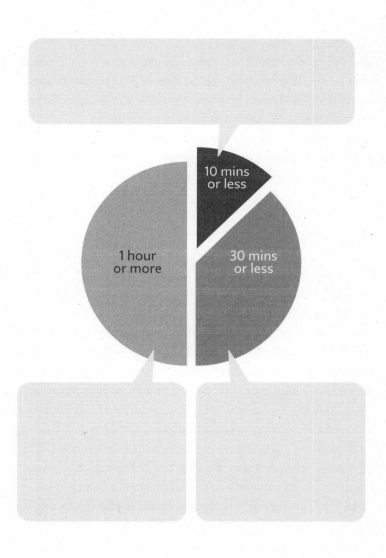

As a minimum, do one thing every week from each section.

Tip: You can add one of these to your checklist at the end of the book, which is also available to download at www.penguin.co.uk/mindfulmenopause.

Once you have created your own foundation for self-care and loving connection, you can begin to create a circle of people around you that can help you on days when you need support most. It may be from within your family, or it may be within your friendship groups, community or even colleagues.

Knowing where that support is, and confidently asking for it when you need it, can strengthen that circle of connection and love that will carry you forward.

A supportive partner

Some partners assume, based on their knowledge of menopause, that it's all down to hormones. Some may think, 'This is how it is going to be from now on,' instead of seeing it as a transition that will adjust and settle over time. Not always, but often, their understanding of this time in a woman's life is very limited.

If you are in the midst of a menopausal transition, you may have barely begun to start talking openly about your experience, but talking to your partner about what is happening, how you are feeling, what sort of approaches you are taking and how they can support you, can make a difference to both of you. It may be understanding the biology of menopause, through to the impact it may make on your sexual relationship. If you are having an unexpected dip in your libido, exploring ways to maintain intimacy with your partner may be a way to keep your physical connection strong. Bank some oxytocin hugs! See Chapter 13 for more about sex and libido.

In many times of transition, if you are in a partnership, you are both existing in a transitional phase. It may not affect your partner physically or psychologically in the same way as you, but they will still be having their own but different experience. They may try to help, or even fix what you are going through . . . but your partner can't fix it, because there is nothing to be fixed.

As you rise to meet your journey, they can walk beside you, being a listener and a non-judgemental observer. They can hold your hand, and offer you love and solidarity, but they cannot take your experience away. They may not always agree with the choices you make, but they can learn to support you in what feels right for you.

Broadly speaking, there are three different roles a supportive partner can provide:

The practical partner thinks about what they can do to practically support you. It may be helping you find ways to cool the bedroom down, or create a retreat in your home; encouraging your goals by walking or exercising with you, or looking after children to give you some me-time. Or, if they love cooking, whipping up some nutritious meals.

The proactive partner might be curious about perimenopause and learn from you – understanding how it affects you, physically and emotionally. Listening to your experiences and needs, and reading your Menopause Plan (see page 197) to learn how you want to approach it, are some ways your partner can be proactive.

The mindful partner is free of judgement. When you are angry and frustrated, they listen and don't make it all about themselves.

They accept and meet your experience with loving kindness and give you space to be who you need to be.

EXERCISE 41: BRINGING YOUR PARTNER UP TO SPEED

At www.penguin.co.uk/mindfulmenopause you can print off the exercise below and personalise it, adding to the different roles to make it your own. It can be a useful guide especially in particularly tough times and a helpful way to give feedback too; if your partner has done something that really helped, let them know. Even if it's a tiny gesture or act of kindness, you can choose to show gratitude for it and write it down, or tell them it 'really helped when . . .' It may not have been obvious in the moment, but on reflection you may realise it made a difference.

Mothering and menopause

If you became a mother later in life, or you have had an early menopause, your children may be quite young; or you may have an adolescent or be an empty nester. Each stage of mothering and menopause brings with it challenges and opportunity.

Whatever age your children are, there is a saying that you might find useful: 'Just one part of your family has to practise mindfulness for the rest of the family to be mindful.'

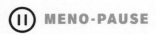 MENO-PAUSE

Being a mother can be tough enough without perimenopause to contend with as well. By cultivating a daily practice of

174

Mindful menopause partner

Practical partner

Practical things that make a difference

Proactive partner

What you need to know about menopause and me!

Compassionate partner

How to support me

It really helped when you....

mindfulness, whether that is starting the day with a waking meditation (see page 92) or a sitting meditation, or consciously taking mindful moments (see page 21) throughout the day, you can start to respond instead of reacting to tinderbox moments.

Self-care and sharing are ways to build a positive and loving connection with your children.

If your children are younger:

- Find time for self-care so you can empty yourself of stress.
- Take mindful walks (see page 281) with your children.
- Find connection and support with friends and family.
- Talk to your partner and your children, however young they are, about how you feel.
- Use the sleep download as often as you can, since sleep can be disrupted more.
- Use your Calm Breath (see page 45).
- Bank those oxytocin hugs from your children!

If you have teens:

- Self-care: are there joint activities you can do with your teen, such as going on a spa day or playing a sport together?
- Talk to your teens about mindfulness and why you are doing it – they may find it helpful too.
- Nurture connections outside your family when your children are able to be left alone for longer.
- Use your Calm Breath (see page 45) in moments when you are clashing with your teen.
- Talk to your teen about menopause – their response might pleasantly surprise you.

- Learn to let go of things that you can't control – choose your battles!

In a home where there are lots of hormones flying around, adjustment and change is happening for everyone. There may be restlessness and emotional discomfort (theirs and yours), which can feel overwhelming. Things can quickly escalate, and it can be hard to be the mother you want to be, or you know you can be, in those moments.

When overwhelm happens, or when you feel anxious, frustrated and angry, these connections can become frayed. Whether you choose to talk to your children about what's happening or not, being open about your feelings is the path to connection. Create a space for open dialogue and don't be afraid to be vulnerable – this can deepen trust and build empathy. You may find that your children start to respond in a supportive way if you tell them you are feeling tired, angry or frustrated and let them know what you need in that moment. By doing this, you can invite them to share what they are experiencing too.

'There are still times when I lose it, exasperated by the mess, by the way everything I own is up for grabs, by the way I'm made to feel so old and boring beside her vibrant youth and beauty – what menopausal woman wouldn't? But there are also immense new pleasures to be gained from watching her blossom into her own woman, full of confidence, ambition and kindness. As I feel my mental horizons constricting with age, I need her to challenge me with the vibrant, passionate idealism of youth. I can perhaps be reminded to stay young at heart.'

Kate Figes

It can be painful if your teenager is going through a tough time but doesn't want your help, especially when you also feel dysregulated. Sometimes you may feel impatient and frustrated wanting to fix things for your child because the feelings are so uncomfortable. Learning to sit in discomfort and connect in a loving way can help you to manage overwhelm, and also give your child the support and space that they need by building a deep unconscious connection. This simple meditation in the next exercise, taught to me by my mother, is something that I do regularly with my boys.

EXERCISE 42: SENDING AND RECEIVING MEDITATION

If your child is angry and upset and doesn't want to talk, and you are feeling overwhelmed as well, it can be tough. You are both going through something. Doing a sending and receiving meditation is powerful. You don't have to be sitting in the same room to do this – your child can be up in their room or even out of the house.

- Just notice where you are sitting or standing and take a deep Calm Breath (see page 45). Take a few deep breaths until you notice your shoulders soften and any tension leave your body. You can close your eyes or keep them open.

- Rest the palm of your hand on your chest where it is comfortable, perhaps just above your heart. Gently smile, breathing tenderness down into your heart. Notice how your heart space feels.

- Imagine a little cloud in front of your heart that can absorb uncomfortable feelings, such as hurt, anger and pain.

- With your next breath in, imagine breathing any of your child's hurt, anger or discomfort in through the cloud and as you breathe out imagine sending love and healing to your child.

- Continue to do this as the discomfort begins to get less and less until it has disappeared.

- Sit in your heart space for a few more breaths, noticing how you are feeling now and, in this stillness, imagine sending the message that you want to send to your child.

Learn from your children

Your children can support you with their imagination, curiosity and passion for life. Engaging in learning new things is great for your brain as well. Join them in conversation, learn new things and be interested in their lives and their views. Learning something completely new can support brain plasticity (see page 93) and engaging in challenging debate supports your memory and brain function.

'I put myself into older parent mode, and stopped worrying about being the "cool Mum". It was a different place – somehow I didn't worry so much and it improved my relationship with the children to let go of expectations.

Although menopause was a difficult emotional journey this made it a lot easier for me and for them.'

Rachael

Family and friends

You may have strong and supportive family relationships. Your own mother may be able to support and guide you, and you may be able to learn from her experience, or perhaps you have sisters and cousins who are going through menopause at a similar time in a similar way to you. You may find that you can build a strong shared connection as you move through this experience.

Friends are the people that you can talk to, laugh with and cry with. Different friends will meet different needs in you. Some will be quiet and reflective; others you can let your hair down with; others you can confide in. Many of them will be going through similar experiences. Find your village, your tribe, the ones you connect with.

If you have found it harder to keep a connection going because life has just been very busy with family, can you start building those relationships again? Is this a time for reconnection?

Community

You can find support in your community in the form of membership at a sports club, or a class you attend weekly, or perhaps by volunteering. Helping others can give you a sense of community and well-being that is heart-opening and joyful. At this time in your life, there may be more opportunities opening up to do this.

Workplace

If you spend most of your week at work, your well-being may be dependent on the environment that you work in and the people you work with. Menopause hasn't been well supported in the workplace and it appears to be one of the last workplace taboos. Rather than be open about the way menopause is affecting their working life, women often change jobs, go part-time or even retire if they are able to. Happily, things are changing and more than ever before workplace support for women experiencing menopause is growing.

Trade unions are now becoming more involved and more progressive, and companies are recognising the impact of menopause on their workforce, exploring policies that address not just the physical aspects of menopause, but also wider aspects of peer support, openness, well-being and absence days.

In 2019, The British Medical Association (BMA) surveyed nearly 2,000 menopausal women working as doctors. Ninety per cent said it impacted their working lives, of those only 15 per cent had discussed this with their manager; 48 per cent wanted to, but did not feel comfortable. That's nearly half of women unable to talk to a manager either because of embarrassment, worry about feeling vulnerable in their job, or fear of bullying and harassment.

To get the support you need, you may need to ask for it. Can you be a pioneer in your workplace? If there is poor ventilation, or it is too hot, request a fan or a seat near a window. Access to toilet facilities is crucial for women that have heavy periods and flooding – is this something that you are able to discuss? If you are in job where you are standing for a long time it may cause discomfort in the joints. This may be easily resolved by thinking creatively about mixing up standing and seated work, depending on your job.

Nothing changes unless we talk about it and many other women may thank you for it. Starting a peer support group internally may be something that you can do easily so you are in it together. Contact your union and see if you can get support from them – the TUC and GMB are doing work around this and you can download toolkits and checklists from their websites. Recommendations include having uniforms with natural fibres, providing water, access to fans, a well-ventilated room, regular rest and being able to report absence due to menopause as sick days.

> 'It's been a normal part of conversation between my peer groups forever, but it's hush hush in the workplace as we can't speak about it or we'll be judged. These things that have been hidden, who have they been hidden from? Men. Has it now become more understood because women are in leadership roles?'
>
> Shelly

As well as having support from your colleagues, you can learn to introduce micro-mindfulness into your day to help your mind and body rest. Punctuating your day with these moments is shown to enhance creativity and be energising. Use your Calm Breath (see page 45) at your desk, before you go into a meeting, or even when you are in a meeting. Aim to do five Mindful Moments (see page 21) a day or one an hour. If you need to, set a reminder on your phone.

EXERCISE 43: CONFIDENCE BREATH

If you need a confidence boost, try this quick visualisation:

- Make yourself comfortable somewhere and use your Calm Breath (see page 45).

- When you feel your shoulders soften, imagine sinking into your Hypnosis Cloud (see page 49).

- Just rest in there for a moment and invite your mind to recall a time when you have felt really confident at work in the past.

- When that comes into your mind, notice all the details.

- Notice that feeling of confidence; it may be a feeling in your body somewhere. Give it a colour.

- With each breath in, breathe in that colour.

- Play it like a film from the beginning of the moment to the end.

- Do this three times.

Each time you need confidence at work, use this breath, breathing your colour of confidence in and breathing out any anxiety.

EXERCISE 44: WHO'S ON YOUR MENOPAUSE TEAM?

Use the illustration overleaf to think about who is on your team. Think about the friends or colleagues that meet some of these aspects of support. Write their names down and a way to contact them, so you can get in touch quickly

Who's in your team?

Someone
who makes
me laugh

Someone who
I can rant at

Someone who I can
do a woman's circle with

Someone
whose shoulder
I can cry on

Someone who
will give me a hug

Someone who
makes me
feel loved

Someone I can
exercise with

when you need to. You can also download this illustration as a **PDF** at www.penguin.co.uk/mindfulmenopause.

Summary

Support begins with you! Make time for self-care, open conversations with those around you. Use your circle of self-care to create a sound foundation for support. Ask for support if you need it and connect with others that are having a similar experience. Build your team, with you at the centre and find ways to maximise your oxytocin through love and connection.

9

Setting Your Intention for
a Positive Menopause

Midlife: when the Universe grabs your shoulders
and tells you 'I'm not f-ing around, use the gifts
you were given.'

Dr Brené Brown from her blog, *The Midlife*

This chapter is really one giant exercise! It is time to chart your course and set your compass to decide what sort of experience you want to have. Now you've changed your filter to absorbing positive messages about menopause and started to address stress in your life, you can start to write your story. Taking the step to let go of other people's stories can feel liberating – your experience is not defined by anyone else's expectations. As you let go of these, you create a space within you from which curiosity can emerge, both of yourself as you grow through this experience and of your changing perspectives of the world around you. A gentle exploration of experience can give you the opportunity to align yourself with your intention to have a positive experience as you move into a new chapter of your life.

'I set myself positive intentions for
midlife and beyond.'

You have a blank page in front of you full of opportunity to allow an experience that feels right for you. Whether you are in your 40s and starting to inform yourself, or in the thick of it, it's always a good time to write down how you wish to experience this time in life, and beyond.

In the midst of change and upheaval, finding the space to sit down, ground yourself in the moment and think of a longer-term plan may seem impossible. Yet, being able to reflect on how you wish to experience menopause, and putting intentions in place to support that, can help guide you in those moments when it feels like you are in a fog and can't think what to do.

It can help to think of any goals or intentions you set as a north star – not as destinations, but as orientations. They will help you find the path that is right for you.

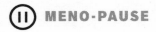 **MENO-PAUSE**

But first, let's start with you!

You are not average, but unique and powerful

You are unique, so your physical experience of perimenopause will be different from everyone else's. From the moment you were born you have lived an extraordinary life, woven together with the stories of your experiences. Some stories may have been wonderful, some may not, but they are a kaleidoscope of experience that form a beautiful pattern. At this moment in time, globally there are around 25 million women every year who are experiencing it with you. Although your experience is your own, you are not in this alone.

Choice is power, and how much you take ownership of your choices can affect your experience in the moment and going forward. This is especially true in menopause when such powerful feelings begin to emerge around disempowerment; it can be a struggle to find your feelings in a society or medical system that doesn't always support the whole woman.

'I feel like I did when I was pregnant – the rest of the world is telling me I am doomed and "just you wait" and "you think you can manage on natural herbs alone? Haha" And I'm quietly in the corner apologising for having the audacity to think that I might rock this woman-lark. Or at least that I might survive it unscathed or un-drugged. I'm using it as an opportunity to do things I've not done before – speak up, trust my intuition, give fewer f*cks, take care of me.'

Mia

I encourage you to start implementing lifestyle changes as early as you can and to read, read, read – read books that you gravitate towards, and some you may not. Something may speak to you that hasn't before. Stretch your understanding of this time beyond your comfort zone and talk to other women. True, no one will quite have the same experience as you, but you can begin to form an idea of what feels right for you as you start to write your Menopause Plan and set your intentions. You may discover that you start to connect with changes to your body and mind more intuitively and begin to notice patterns.

> 'As I am learning about my body, I
> am learning about my choices.'

Although menopause is a powerful transition, it is still very medicalised, when in truth it can be one of the most profound spiritual experiences for women. Very often the approach is HRT or 'natural'. It's not as simple as taking HRT or not taking HRT – there is a whole other dimension that is mostly unexplored.

When I hear the words 'menopause fog', I don't think of the brain. I think of the medical fog that clouds spiritual growth at this time. There are statistics about the average time that perimeno-pause starts, how long it lasts, what 'symptoms' women have. This medical model of menopause gives a set of cultural expecta-tions of how it will be, but this may not fit for you and it might feel uncomfortable to be squeezed into a box that just isn't right.

Your three intelligence centres

You have three intelligence centres that help you to access all the information your body and mind has when making deci-sions, setting intentions or planning aspects of life. These are:

- Your head – what you think about it
- Your heart – your emotions around it
- Your gut – your feelings around it

These three centres are in constant communication with each other and your decision-making is a result of the unconscious exchange of information shared between them. Learning how to bring these together and balance your head, heart and gut when it comes to decision-making can help you make choices that impact positively on your life.

> 'I let my mind hear my heart and
> my mouth speak its words.'

There is some evidence to suggest that in the years running up to menopause your decision-making balance becomes weighted towards your heart and gut. Isn't that wonderful? This can be liberating day to day – following your heart and gut can feel so joyful. However, before making really big decisions that could be life-changing you may wish to learn to consciously take time to seek a balanced input from each one of your decision-making centres.

When working on your Menopause Plan, whether it's a daily intention or a monthly intention, listen to those three centres – feel where they pull you, feel where they repel you. Your gut instinct is powerful. It may be easy, or it may take you time, but your inner voice needs to be heard. That voice will grow stronger during the years approaching menopause – as if it's saying, 'Hey! Listen to me'.

> 'As I move into a new chapter of
> my life, I align with positive
> intention.'

Tip: if you have a decision to make in the moment, even if it's something small like turning on the television, sit and think about it. Imagine your analytical response, then put your hand on your heart and ask which emotion is connected with it. Then switch your attention to your gut and notice what your gut is saying. You can give each part a percentage based on how much of a role they take in your decision-making.

EXERCISE 45: CONNECTING WITH YOUR INTUITION

For the next week, or even just for today, notice the spontaneous subtle responses that you may not normally be aware of when you make a choice, even a little one. It may be your response when the doorbell rings, or you get a text message; it may be when someone asks you if you want something. Listen to your whole-body response in those moments. If something doesn't feel right to you, there may be a sense of heaviness or a pressure on your chest, or a tightness in your throat or in your stomach. Sometimes making a decision makes you feel lighter and energised; sometimes you may not feel anything at all, just a sense that you do or don't want to do something.

Make a note of your responses in your journal and reflect on them when you feel drawn to it. As you do, you may notice a more conscious connection with your deeper knowledge evolving.

Now let's get started with setting your menopause goals, your intention for a framework within with you that can flow and grow. Think about what you want from this next chapter in your life, bringing your knowledge, experience, instincts and desires to the table. Your story is no average story – this is your new chapter, your experience moving forward. It's time to start writing it.

Your menopause goals

If you were sitting in front of me right now in a hypnotherapy session, the first question I would ask you is, 'If you were to have a positive menopause, how would it look?' When thinking about your menopause goals, avoid writing how you *don't* want to be and instead think how you *do* want to be. Your goals have to be positive, achievable and realistic so that you can start to integrate them into your daily life.

As perimenopause can happen over a long period of time, it's helpful to break these down into:

1. Long-term goals
2. Medium-term goals, which are monthly and annually
3. Short-term goals, which are weekly and daily

An annual goal may be going away by yourself for a weekend. Shorter-term goals may be waking up energised on weekday mornings.

Then you need to think of the actions that underpin these goals. How are you going to change your behaviour and actions? This is where many of the tools in the book come in, especially those in the experience-specific chapters in the second section of the book.

If your weekly goal is to wake up in the mornings feeling energised and looking forward to the day ahead, it may be that you commit to doing some of the tools in the sleep chapter (see page 203); for example, the morning movement meditation or waking affirmations. If your goal is to have a weekend away by yourself once a year, make steps to research and book it. My sister lives in Sydney and I hadn't visited her for nearly 16 years (the age of my eldest son). I worried about how my family would manage without me. Someone said, 'Just book the ticket. You want to go to see your sister. Book the ticket, the rest will work itself out.' And it did.

Sometimes you just have to set things in motion so that the doors begin to open. Your mind has an extraordinary way of aligning your experience with actions and intentions. The filter that we talked about on page 136 has a big role to play in this. When you set an intention and you work towards that intention, your filter starts to change and suddenly opportunities that align with your intention are revealed to you. It may seem coincidental or serendipitous, but it's your magic that is making this happen. There are limitless opportunities that will present themselves when you allow yourself to connect with your deeper intention to experience menopause in the way that you want to. Make menopause what you will.

EXERCISE 46: COMMITTING TO YOUR GOALS

Once you've thought about the goals you want to achieve, write them in your journal; they can be adapted and changed at any point, but by writing them down they will become more real. You might want to write your short-term goals on sticky notes and place them somewhere that you will see them regularly.

EXERCISE 47: BE GUIDED BY YOUR INNER WISE WOMAN

Imagine that you are the woman you want to be during menopause or post-menopause. Consider her attitude, her hobbies, how she looks. Find your role models, look at the women around you, perhaps older people with qualities that you respect. What qualities do you value in older women? When you were a child was there an older woman or a person in your life who made you feel loved, warm, comfortable and safe? Was there someone who looks great, or has achieved something amazing? Bring all the qualities together into one person, into you. Close your eyes and imagine yourself in ten years' time, maybe 15, standing in front of this person. Imagine asking them what they did, how they did it, what new habits did they have to adapt to? You can consult with the wise woman in you whenever you feel at a crossroads or want a bit of motivation.

You may want to use your journal to make a note of this or keep a notebook just to track thoughts and feelings that arise in relation to your goals. You may find that a question may not be answered in the moment you ask, but that the answer will emerge through dreams or even pop into your thoughts unexpectedly.

Tip: Spend an afternoon pulling together words, images or photos that you want to identity with the wise woman in you and stick them into a page in your journal, so you can reflect and take counsel from that part of you whenever you feel the need.

Give your goals a power boost!

You can power-charge your goals by visualising yourself doing them. I love micro-goals and use them all the time in my work and on myself. When you imagine yourself achieving something, whether it's getting out of bed when your alarm goes off, completing a project, or reaching a target at the gym, it is evidenced that by living your goal internally, it happens more easily externally. If you need to remind yourself of how visualisation works, go back to the section on page 50.

EXERCISE 48: VISION BOARD IT

Vision boards or manifestation boards are becoming more popular and are a great way to bring your goals into your mind's awareness. They are particularly effective during this life stage when you are likely to be feeling more creative. Hormonal changes and shifts can radically enhance the more creative parts of your brain, so anything that involves expressing your creativity can get really great results.

- Grab a piece of card A4 or bigger.

- Find some images, either from magazines or online, of older women who embody qualities you love.

- Gather some affirmations and positive words.

- Find other things to make your board creative . . .

Now create a board of how you want to approach this stage of your life. Use images, words, write affirmations. Think of things you want to do, people you want to surround yourself with.

When you are finished, stick it up somewhere you will see it a lot, or photograph it and use it as a screen saver.

Tip: Remember to revisit your goals on a regular basis. As you start to act and engage in achieving your goals, you may start to discover knowledge and information that is still aligned with your purpose to have a calm and confident menopause and you may wish to write new ones. Imagine this book is a springboard. Like many other people who have read my books, you may find that it's the beginning of an incredible journey into a world you didn't even know existed!

Writing your Menopause Plan

Twenty years ago, it wasn't commonplace to write a birth plan; women just went in and gave birth, usually in a hospital. Now, writing a birth plan is something nearly every pregnant woman does. Why? Because more and more women are learning the importance of their birth experience and that one approach does not suit everyone. This movement is being driven by women who have discovered that the transition from maiden to mother can be transformative and empowering, not something to be anxious about. Moreover, ownership of this experience through decision-making cultivates a deep sense of well-being and awareness of their capacity to grow into motherhood.

I don't feel that this has happened for menopause, but there is change afoot and you are right in the middle of the next powerful transition awakening. There is a huge groundswell of voices – women wanting to own, know and meet their experience of menopause fully as they move into the next stage of their lives. You can be stylish, sexy, reflective, healthy, spiritually connected; you can be whatever you want. But planning is a big part of this.

Have your A plan – dream big. If you could wave a magic wand, what do your plans encompass?

My Menopause Plan

It's useful to do your research before you write your plan, especially if there are aspects that you are unsure about. Integrating your values (see pages 152–153), as well as knowledge from this book and other resources, can help you to craft a plan to refer to when you need to make a decision about your well-being, whether it's physical, emotional or spiritual. If you are able to, sharing this with a partner or friend may be helpful for added support and encouragement.

Think of what you include in your plan as preferences that are open to change. In a time of upheaval, creating movement and fluidity of choice can engender a feeling of being in control. When a plan falls apart, it can feel like failure, but there is no failure when it is a preference; only a gentle holding of your wishes for an experience that echoes your soul. Being able to adapt and alter your preferences while still staying true to your values, will help you feel connected to your experience in an empowering way.

(II) MENO-PAUSE

I've written some examples of what you might include in your plan below to get you started. Think about what you really want, how you want to navigate this stage in your life, what you want to open up to, and what you absolutely don't want.

I want to approach my menopause with patience, allowing it to unfold, with all its up and downs in the time that it needs to take.

It can take time to pass through menopause – for some it will be longer than for others. Whatever the duration, it will almost certainly be up and down. Some days the waves will toss you around and it'll be harder to hold on and other days it will feel peaceful. Learning to put yourself first, and to cultivate patience is to show loving kindness to the part of you that is adapting and growing. Having this in your preferences is a reminder to think about the tools and techniques in this book and to find places where patience has the space to rest tenderly in your body and mind.

I don't want to medicate/I do want to medicate/I want to try complementary approaches first if I need some help.
Often medication is offered and it may be something you want, or you don't want. Listen to your gut feeling. As mentioned earlier in the chapter, your journey to menopause and beyond is completely unique to you. Many women I speak to say that they don't want to take something unless they have to, and if they were struggling, they would rather try a complementary approach first. I'd recommend exploring some of the resources included in the back of this book (see page 311), so you get a balanced view. I always advise my clients to make a decision not from a place of fear or worry, but from a place of peace and power.

I want an area in my home I can retreat to, and reflect and relax in.
Think about what your retreat space will look like (see page 151). Write this down as part of you plan and set time aside to create it.

On days when I feel overwhelmed I want time to myself/positive encouragement/hugs!
Your partner might find it helpful to understand what you are experiencing, with a view to supporting you in the way that is

consistent with your chosen approach. Partners and friends can often fall foul to the same cultural narratives and may not think twice, often using humour to try to smooth things over. Jokes like 'Oh, you're so menopausal' trip out of people's mouths sometimes.

I'll be expanding my horizons by exploring something new, such as volunteering/singing/tennis/yoga.
Include these ideas in your plan. As I've said before, this is a great time to learn something new and a reminder to yourself that this can be a time for expansion. Try a few activities out before settling on what lifts your soul.

I want people around me who are positive/encouraging/funny/ supportive/uplifting.
Think about who in your life reflects what you need during this transition. Return to the exercise on building your team on page 83.

Summary

It may seem like you have a lot to think about and to do after reading this chapter, but I hope you see it as exciting and fun. Setting your intention for a positive menopause and putting a plan in place can help you to make choices that support your well-being and quality of life.

PART 3

What You Can Do About It

10

Feeling Rested

Innocent sleep. Sleep that soothes away all our
worries. Sleep that puts each day to rest. Sleep that
relieves the weary labourer and heals hurt minds.
Sleep, the main course in life's feast, and the most
nourishing.

William Shakespeare, *Macbeth*

Clients often ask me, 'Will hypnosis help me sleep more?'
The short answer is, 'Yes,' but it's not as straightforward
as responding to a hypnosis suggestion along the lines of, 'You
will go into a deep and restful sleep for eight hours each and
every night.'

There is a plethora of information in the media about sleep
that can cause confusion and concern – with the suggestion
that if we fall short of the right amount and type of sleep it will
adversely impact our life. These messages, and most of the
research, don't take menopause into account – the gender
health gap (see page 85) means that we need to look at the
nature of sleeplessness and sleep during menopause in a different way.

During perimenopause it is normal for sleep patterns
to change. Recognising what's changing and why, and understanding what you can do about it, can help you adapt more

easily to those shifting patterns without being anxious about 'not getting enough sleep'. Remember too, that menopause is not always the underlying issue. Some medical conditions lead to poor sleep, so if your pattern significantly changes and you don't really identify with any of the triggers in this chapter, it may be worth having a chat with your doctor.

Change begins with seeing things in a different way, so in this chapter I invite you to put anything you know about sleep aside and start to explore a variety of approaches to feeling rested during perimenopause and beyond.

Sleeplessness or insomnia?

Among those experiencing perimenopause will be a number of people who have had sleep issues all their lives. This is known as chronic insomnia and it's extremely tough – it's also hard to talk about as others often don't understand how debilitating it can be. Insomnia is a sleep disorder that is defined as having three or more sleepless nights a week over a period of one month or more; often it causes significant distress and difficulty at work and at home. Depression and anxiety can also be a result of ongoing lack of sleep.

Being able to distinguish between perimenopausal sleeplessness and clinical insomnia can help you to find practical solutions and create healthy patterns around sleep to support this stage of your life. One of the biggest triggers I see for long-term sleep problems beginning in perimenopause arises from disrupted sleep patterns, because of physical disturbances such as hot flushes. A few disrupted nights may create fear and anxiety around sleep, and we know from research that this can lead to a cycle of anxiety and sleeplessness.

While medication is often prescribed for insomnia, evidence shows that psychological therapies, particularly Cognitive Behavioural Therapy (CBT), hypnosis and mindfulness can be more effective in the long term. Hypnosis and mindfulness are particularly good at reducing anxiety, alertness, rumination and mental overactivity – all known to be contributing factors for poor sleep.

In perimenopause, instead of considering HRT doctors often prescribe sleep medication or antidepressants. HRT can also have a benefit, principally because it can reduce hot flushes and joint pains in the night, both of which can disturb sleep, and it can also reduce anxiety. Very rarely are women offered a psychological therapy for sleep issues, despite the evidence of its effectiveness. Some of my clients have chosen to take medication alongside psychological therapies with the intention of coming off the medication once they feel they have more knowledge and understanding of their personal sleep patterns.

Changes in sleep patterns can give you insight into your thoughts and feelings and what's happening physically – they can be a 'wake-up call' to change something in your life, whether it's around diet, exercise, work, home or something bigger and more life-changing.

'I let go of any worry around sleep
and learn to give my mind and
body the rest it needs.'

You are not an insomniac

How we talk about insomnia is very interesting. The word 'insomnia' actually comes from the Latin for sleepless, but in today's culture it is weighed down with so much more meaning.

Clients often tell me they are 'an insomniac'. I'm interested in their use of language as it tells me that the person has identified their self with insomnia; it's part of who they are. This is very different from a person experiencing a run of sleepless nights. Remember, you are not the experience or the behaviour; you are having that experience in that moment in time. It's easier to change an experience than change yourself isn't it?

Have you ever heard of 'sleep misperception'? Research shows some people can be asleep without realising it. It can feel as if they are consciously aware, yet scans show their brainwaves slowing down into a theta state of rest. We don't know why this happens yet, but it's a growing area of research.

EXERCISE 49: SLEEP AFFIRMATIONS

You can redefine your experience of sleep and rest using affirmations. Positive affirmations and suggestions are shown to improve sleep. Here are some examples, but try also writing your own:

- 'As I rest my mind, I rest my body.'

- 'My mind is quiet as I feel relaxed and comfortable in my bed.'

- 'I am at ease as my body settles into sleep.'

- 'If I wake in the night I will return to sleep because my body knows how to sleep.'

Write your own here or in your journal:

_____

_____

_____

You can also start to use the phrase, 'I had a sleepless night' instead of saying, 'My insomnia was really bad last night.'

Connecting with your sleep pattern

Everyone has different sleep patterns, and during menopause it's about finding a regular one that works for you. Your patterns may have shifted during your life, perhaps due to sleep disruptions from children or illness, or if you have ever been a carer for someone in your family.

Patterns are known to shift at times when there have been significant hormonal transitions. For example, when you were an adolescent you would have probably benefitted from going to bed later and waking up later; if you have teenagers, you will have been reminded of that pattern. If you have had children, you'll be familiar with the disrupted patterns in the early years, which can take a long to time to readjust to.

Then during perimenopause shifts start to happen again; in fact, as you become older, you may find that you need less sleep and that your pattern changes again. Imagine seeing this from a distance as an observer of the rhythm of life – the waves of sleep adjusting to a moving tide. Being alert to your own personal sleep pattern at different times in your life will help you to see it as an impermanent pattern.

Research shows that the average amount of sleep for an older adult is between seven to nine hours a night; many people have the figure of eight hours fixed in their minds as the optimum amount of sleep, but as with everything there are outliers. Research shows that 1 per cent of the population are able to function very well on less than five hours. What's important is finding what works for you and discovering your own unique 'sleep window' or 'windows'.

Some people sleep through the night, for example from 11pm–6am; other people have sleep windows, perhaps falling asleep at 10pm, waking up at 2am for an hour or so, then going back to sleep from 3–6am.

Can you shift your focus from the hours you think you should be sleeping to discovering which pattern of sleep helps you to wake up feeling refreshed or to function well throughout the day? What's more important? The number of hours you sleep or whether you feel able to go about your normal day free of fatigue?

EXERCISE 50: KNOW YOUR SLEEP WINDOW

Forget what people say about eight hours sleep. Think about what you would typically need to feel rested. What time do you start to feel sleepy and go to bed, and what time do you typically wake up? Close your eyes and bring yourself into a state of light relaxation using the Hypnosis Cloud (see page 49). Then bring a recent night into your mind when you slept and woke up feeling rested. Notice where you were, what was in your environment, what your pattern was and how you felt.

Now imagine taking elements of that experience from that night into a future night. It may be this week, next week or even tonight. Play that film over in your mind five times, so your mind knows that this is something that you wish to do, and it becomes familiar with it. Over time, if you find that your sleep window starts to shift, then do this again. You can help your mind to reset itself and recognise its most restorative sleep window at regular times during perimenopause and the years following menopause.

Mindful sleep hygiene

I'm sure you've heard of sleep hygiene, and if you have ever had a run of bad sleep it's usually the first thing that someone suggests, perhaps to your annoyance! However, I'm hoping that the following aspects of sleep hygiene that are particularly relevant during perimenopause will be helpful, along with the section on how mindfulness or hypnosis can help to turn this into regular and unconscious behaviour.

Smoking

The link between smoking and sleep issues is well established. Giving up smoking can have huge benefits to your well-being during menopause, but withdrawal of nicotine can cause temporary sleep disruption.

Hypnosis: I've used hypnosis to help hundreds of clients stop smoking, and I always prepare them for sleep disruption. If you are ready and motivated to stop, a session or few with a hypno-therapist can really give you the boost you need. If you can't get to a hypnotherapist, you can listen to a download or do an online course.

Sleep scheduling

There is compelling evidence that keeping a regular sleep sched-ule is one of the best ways to help insomnia and improve sleep quality. This means going to bed and waking up at the same time *every* day. Even though it may be tempting to sleep in at the weekend or when on holiday, keep to your sleep schedule.

When on holiday, introduce other restful activities, many of which are in this book. The benefit of being on holiday is that you can make a commitment to a sleep schedule for the length of time you are away and see how that is for you. Your sleep schedule may change during perimenopause, so if you feel you are waking up very early, try going to bed an hour later for a week to see if it makes a difference.

Hypnosis: Therapies such as CBT and cognitive hypnosis take sleep scheduling into account during treatment for sleep issues with good results. By understanding and creating a strong connection to your sleep window (see page 208), it can be easier to stick to your schedule. Use positive suggestions such as, 'Tomorrow I am going to wake up and get out of bed at [whichever time you have chosen] and I am going to go to bed at [again, whichever time you have chosen].'

Mental well-being

General day-to-day anxiety or specific events that cause anxiety can trigger a bad night's sleep, and lead to continuing sleep disruption if the anxiety persists. This can be any-thing from being overloaded at work, being anxious about getting on a plane, concern about a medical appointment or waiting for your children's exam results. Being able to let go of those things that are causing anxiety at the end of the day by emptying your mind onto a piece of paper can be helpful.

If you have a busy day, perhaps balancing work and home life, maybe caring for children or elderly parents, the moment your head hits the pillow may be the first moment you have had to yourself that day. Your brain may want to use this time to start processing things that you haven't had a chance to think about. Equally, if there is something that is worrying you it can be a time that you find yourself ruminat-ing on it.

Mindfulness: Mindfulness is great for reducing stress. By learning to reflect on the day and let it go, your mind and body can let go of feelings it is holding onto. Try doing The Spotlight exercise (see page 111) for ten minutes at the end of the day.

Hypnosis: Daily hypnosis visualisation, positive suggestion and guided audio tracks can help to process stress and change your response to situations you may find stressful. Letting go of worries or things that you are ruminating over can be done quickly and easily with a simple hypnosis track. 🎧 Listen to the Letting Go audio on page 26.

Tip: As you walk towards your bedroom at night, give yourself permission to leave anything that may be troubling you out-side the door. Imagine a magical wall that any worries and stress can't pass through.

Light and noise disturbances

Using light to create a rhythm when going to bed and waking up can enhance your quality of sleep. As it gets towards bedtime, start to dim your lights – this will be a sure sign to your body that you are winding down for sleep. Make sure that any devices that may light up or beep are removed or switched off. When you get up, try to get some daylight perhaps by standing in your garden or on a balcony or by going for a short walk. Make sure that you punctuate your day with sunlight in some way.

Some of my clients are very sensitive to noise in their environment. The good news is that you can learn to integrate those sounds into your falling asleep experience in a beneficial way, using the simple mindfulness technique and hypnosis exercise below.

Mindfulness: By naming the sounds and disturbances in your room, you can start to accept them and let them go. Use The Spotlight exercise on page 111.

Hypnosis: Change what the sounds mean to you. If your partner is snoring, instead of it being a disruption, think of it as something that helps you go to sleep. What do you find reassuring about your partner being there in bed with you? What would it be like for you if they weren't there every night? That may be a different conversation!

EXERCISE 51: SNORING LULLABY

If the sound you find disruptive is your partner snoring, find the positive in them being there and turn it into a positive affirmation: 'Each time I hear my partner snoring, I am . . .'

This may be quite difficult to say at first, especially if you don't believe it, but remember what you learned about affirmations on page 38. You have to say them regularly before you believe in them, and your response starts to change.

You can turn outside noises such as traffic, trains, planes and people coming back from a night out, into something that sends you deeper into sleep. Try an affirmation along the lines of:

'Everything is secure. I am safe in my room and I am ready for sleep.'

Or:

'Every sound [you can choose to add a specific sound] that I hear sends me deeper into sleep and rest, safe in the knowledge that everything is well.'

My clinic is on a busy intercity rail line – and, after years of saying to my clients, 'The sound of the train soothes you and sends you deeper into relaxation,' I moved into a house that backed onto the same line. I found that it didn't bother me at all; in fact, it made me feel deeply relaxed. It's all about perspective, as anyone who has lived under a flight path will be able to tell you!

Movement

The jury is out on whether it is better to exercise in the morning or the evening, so listen to your body and do what feels right for you. Some people say that they are more alert after exercising in the evening, whereas others find that they rest well after exercising after work, or at the end of the day. Research suggests that the link between sleep and exercise is more focused on cognitive arousal, which means that exercise can heighten awareness. What we do know is that some exercise can help you sleep, even taking a short walk around the block during the day can help.

Mindfulness: Try doing a restful sequence of mindful movements such as yoga, or simple stretching at the end of the day before you go to bed.

Hypnosis: Visualise yourself getting up from your desk and going for a walk at lunchtime. Micro-goal visualisations can be brilliant to help motivate you to make daily or even hourly changes! You can visualise putting your shoes on, breathing in the fresh air, the route you are taking, or even that lightness you feel once you have finished.

Food and drink

This one is quite specific to perimenopause and the years that follow menopause. As oestrogen drops, metabolism changes and slows down, so apart from needing less energy, the rate at which you digest food can slow down.

A huge 2019 study with data from over 50,000 women post-menopause over a three-year period showed that the risk of developing insomnia was greater in women who included more sugars in their diet, such as white and brown sugar, syrups, honey and molasses. The risk of developing insomnia was lower in women who ate more whole fruits and vegetables. The suggestion is that a low-GI diet could help with sleep challenges during menopause. Alcohol can also have an impact on sleep and well-being – it's thought that it may increase hot flushes, which at night can be one of the biggest sleep disrupter.

Mindfulness: Eating mindfully can connect you to your body and the food you are eating in a much more meaningful way. Studies show that mindful eating can result in significant changes in weight, eating behaviour and psychological well-being. We'll explore more of this in Chapter 15.

Hypnosis: Hypnotherapy and self-hypnosis are effective approaches to altering attitudes and behaviour towards nutrition. Some habits may be hard to break, for example sugar cravings, but you can do it. The body adapts very quickly, and the results will soon be felt. Often women describe it as a lightness and of feeling more energy. You can find out more in Chapter 15.

Tip: Hydrate in the early part of the day and don't drink too much in the hours before you go to bed. Oestrogen can weaken muscles in the bladder, so reducing pressure on the bladder at night can help you to sleep through much more easily.

Environment

Your sleep environment matters and not just the aspects that you are aware of – unconscious associations have more of an impact than we realise. Creating a space that is private and safe helps your body and mind to wind down. Can you re-create your sleep space so that you feel nurtured, enclosed and comfortable? Close your eyes and think what your ideal bedroom would look and feel like. Think about colours that perhaps make you feel cool, but comfortable. Is your bedding inviting? Have a scent in your room that you associate with being relaxed and calm. Do you feel more able to relax when your room is tidy?

Hypnosis: With conditioning and self-hypnosis, you can create calming associations using smell in your room. This will help your unconscious mind to switch off and slow down as you drift into sleep. Perhaps you can't create your ideal room for practical reasons, but think about why it's your ideal and bring as much of it as you can into your bedroom.

EXERCISE 52: SLEEP SCENT

Using the self-hypnosis skills you've learned, you can create the anchor to a particular smell you find calming and restful. It's a form of conditioning – all you have to do is think of a place where you felt calm, relaxed, safe and then through these steps you link the feeling of being in that place to a scent.

First of all think of your calm place, it may have been on holiday, a place you spent time as a child, or somewhere completely made up! If your place changes during the exercise, that's okay, it may just be your mind shuffling a few around to see which one fits best.

Now follow these steps:

1. Find a smell, an essential oil or similar, that you find restful.
2. Put it nearby on a pillow or a piece of tissue or in a diffuser.
3. Lie down on your bed and make yourself comfortable.
4. Use your Calm Breath (see page 45) until you feel your shoulders soften.

5. Bring your calm place into your mind. Imagine it in detail as if you were there again.
6. Continue to breathe deeply.
7. Repeat this every night for a week.

By practising this exercise regularly, the restful smell will be associated with that feeling of calm in a place where you feel as if you can let go. Putting this scent on in the room when you go to bed will create a calming, restful state at a very deep unconscious level – inviting you into restorative sleep.

Cool it!

This part of sleep hygiene is specific to menopause. Hot flushes are one of the main reasons why sleep is disrupted, but you can minimise them by preparing your environment and reducing stress before you go to bed. Research shows simply having your window open at night can make a big difference. Think about what else you can do practically to cool yourself in the night – perhaps changing your bedding and duvet to something cooler, or wearing different nightwear or nothing at all. If you experience hot flushes, you may want to keep spare nightwear to hand.

Tip: Take seven flannels and soak them in water, maybe with a drop of lavender oil, and then put each one in a freezer bag or similar. Pop them in the freezer. If you are getting a lot of hot flushes, take one out and put it by your bed, so that if you wake you have something that you can use to cool down quickly.

Turning restless sleep into restful nights

Sleeplessness is a very individual experience. Tailoring your environment and winding down well can help you get into a deep sleep quickly, but what if you are someone who wakes in the middle of the night and doesn't get back to sleep?

If you are very alert, and not sleepy at all, move to another room and do something restful. Sometimes it can take a while to feel sleepy again, and that's okay – listen to your body. For people that experience poor sleep and know what fatigue feels like, feeling anxious about not being able to get back to sleep is understandable. When you are worried or anxious, even if that's unconscious, your body releases adrenaline and is on a state of alert. Remember you are a mammal and if you are in a state of alert, your body won't want you to go into a deep sleep. Sleep hormones, such as melatonin, are incompatible with stress hormones – you can't have both at the same time – but rest assured, you can learn how to lower your stress hormones so that your sleep hormones can do what they are able to do in the best way for you.

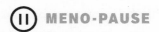 **MENO-PAUSE**

Start to reframe this shift in your sleep pattern as something that you can accept for this day, for this moment in time. For some people it is actually normal to get up at around 4am and sometimes what is 'normal' changes. Before I had children, I would sleep so well, whenever I liked. After having children, I mourned my lack of sleep, and always thought, 'When the kids sleep more, it will go back to normal.' It never returned to the pattern I had pre-children, but I feel rested most of the time. Now moving through perimenopause, my pattern is shifting again.

The truth is there is no normal; there's just the sleep you have in the moment you are in. You can't dwell on the sleep you haven't had or become anxious about the sleep that may be disrupted. You can only focus on what it is right now, and you can choose to rest your mind and be in that space.

Maybe for now this is your sleep schedule. When hormones are in a state of adjustment, you might find that your sleep window shifts and adjusts as well – don't fight it, go with it.

🎧 EXERCISE 53: HYPNOSIS FOR RESTORATIVE SLEEP

This track is available for download (see page 9).

It will help you to lower any stress hormones and bring you into a restful state of mind. You can listen to it before you go to sleep at night, or on waking in the night. It may appear not to be doing anything, but your mind will benefit from the rest you have while you are listening.

During perimenopause higher levels of cortisol may be the reason for sleep changes, such as night waking. Before waking often the body will have a surge of cortisol. You can learn to support these changes in a positive way by practising meditation. Evidence shows that mindfulness-based approaches reduce cortisol levels.

Sleep and rest

As a culture, we place a tremendous amount of value on sleep – the amount of hours, the depth and quality, and so on. But do we ever consider the value of rest? Hypnosis is all about encouraging people to think differently about a situation, to see it in a different and better way. As you read this chapter you may have started to notice your perception shift about how many hours you 'need', or which pattern you 'should' follow.

I invite you to turn your intention to the value of rest. Even if you don't feel like sleeping, you can rest your mind – and your mind will love you for this! Mind-resting can take the form of a mindfulness exercise or a guided meditation, a mindful walk (see page 281) or even a hypnosis session.

Scattered thoughts and a busy mind work your brain to the max, because so many things are being juggled. Taking time during the day to rest your mind can impact positively on the quality of your sleep, but also energise you.

A hypnosis sleep track or a Yoga Nidra meditation, which is a body scan that uses focused attention, are wonderfully relaxing tools for resting or sleeping. They can help you to fall asleep, or simply rest your mind. Research shows that 30 minutes of this type of activity can be the equivalent to three hours of sleep in terms of rest.

Aware that often people only have time for short breaks during the day, a recent study successfully adapted a Yoga Nidra meditation into just 11 minutes, the idea being that it could be integrated into a busy day but still have a significant effect on sleep.

You can also take short pauses throughout the day to recalibrate and ground yourself. Practising a Mindful Moment (see page 21) when you remember can have a significant impact on your well-being. It doesn't matter where you are – whether you are at work, at home, or out and about, you can punctate your day with mindful moments.

🐏 EXERCISE 54: YOGA NIDRA

You can download a short Yoga Nidra meditation (see page 9) for those quick breaks during the day. There is a longer sleep hypnosis track for night-time.

Summary

Throw the textbook on sleep out of the window. Don't think about hours of sleep – think 'How and when I can rest my mind?' Use your Meno-Pauses! Now is the time to notice your sleep window as it shifts and changes. Start to think about sleep hygiene if you haven't before, using some of the tools in this chapter. Use mindfulness throughout your day to help reduce stress hormones and have a go at the hypnosis tool to enhance a feeling of calm and relaxation in the bedroom, as well as reframing those pesky night-time noises into something that helps you instead of hinders you.

11

Hot Flushes and Cool Thoughts

What I would say, which I've said to myself and to girlfriends who've also experienced hot flashes, in particular, is that change is part of being human. We evolve and should not fear that change. You're not alone.

Kim Cattrall

Hot flushes are nearly always the first thing that women talk about when it comes to menopause. There are countless comedy memes of women with beads of sweat coming off them, holding fans up to their faces, or standing in front of an open fridge at 3am. Humour aside, hot flushes can be disruptive and life-changing. They are not 'just a hot sweat'. They can come on suddenly and without warning, like a volcano erupting from deep within and spreading throughout your body. Some women sweat heavily and have to change their clothes or sheets afterwards. If you have had this experience you may think that nothing can help, but I'm here to reassure you that you can find ways to change your experience.

We don't know exactly why hot flushes happen, but all the research suggests that the changes in oestrogen affect the part of the brain, the hypothalamus, that regulates temperature. This area is your thermostat and during menopause it is really sensitive to slight changes in body temperature, so if you are too warm, it can set off a chain of events to cool you down – this results in a hot flush.

'It helps to have a positive mentality. You are not a 'victim'. Just get on with your life and don't let it become an excuse for not living. Find ways to accommodate the effects. I would shower and dress but by the time I got to work, I had to shower again and put on fresh clothes. So, I just accepted that's what I had to do.'

Ellen

Hot flushes can happen anywhere at any time – in a meeting at work, in the supermarket, on a train and during the night. They may even cause the battle of the bed as you vie to be as close as possible to an open window in the middle of winter.

You may never have a hot flush; you may have them infrequently or they may be frequent and distressing. In the earlier stages of menopause, 40 per cent of women have them clustered around their periods, and later in menopause up to 80 per cent will have had an experience of them. Hot flushes tend to be resolved within around five years of them starting.

It's not just heat that the body has trouble regulating; less spoken about but also experienced by some women are cold flushes. As the body is adjusting its temperature after a hot flush seeking to find balance, you may experience chills, especially if you sweat and your clothes or sheets are damp.

Remarkably we know that thoughts can impact on the experience of hot flushes as research shows that up to 40 per cent of women see an improvement when using a placebo. Never underestimate the power of how it is to take control and to feel that you are doing something to make a difference.

'I have the power within me to change my experience.'

In this chapter I've drawn on the experience of women I have worked with and the tools that have worked for them. There is strong evidence to show that hypnotherapy, Cognitive Behavioural Therapy (CBT) and Mindfulness-Based Stress Reduction (MBSR) can significantly reduce or eliminate hot flushes altogether and they are just some of the non-pharmacological treatments that are recommended. One study showed that hypnosis reduced hot flushes by 74 per cent!

I'm going to give you some generic tools and visualisations, but will combine them with a personalised approach so that you can create your own toolbox to reduce or eliminate hot flushes. By doing this, you can supercharge those tools. If you were my client, sitting across the chair from me, I would always start by asking what you already know about hot flushes. Usually, my clients have already done a lot of research and know the small adjustments and changes that they can make. In fact, there is no shortage of suggestions online or in other books.

The reason why talking therapies and mindfulness-based therapies are proven to be so effective is that they help you to design a response that is reflective of your life. My goal is to help you build on what you already know by consolidating your knowledge with the tools in this chapter.

Changing your experience of a hot flush

Whether you have hot flushes or not, if you are perimenopausal you can begin to think about lifestyle changes that will make a difference to your experience of these vasomotor (VSM) aspects of menopause. Stress reduction, sleep and diet can all help you to manage your experience of hot flushes. So far in this book, you've read about the Calm Breath, The Control Room, and using colour visualisations and imagery – all of these techniques can be applied here. Keep them in mind and start to make the connection to those and any hot flushes you may be experiencing in specific situations.

I'm going to structure this loosely around a typical hypnotherapy session. As I'm not actually sitting across from you, listening to your answers, I encourage you to be honest with yourself and write down the best answers you can. You can use your journal to do this as well. You will begin to see a pattern emerge with some ideas of how you can tailor your own approach to hot flushes.

You are going to learn how to:

1. Notice patterns
2. Apply your coping strategies
3. Recognise your triggers
4. Use hypnosis and mindfulness tools

Learning to notice patterns

Have you ever stopped to think about whether there is a pattern to your hot flushes? Are there particular places where they are more frequent? For example, when you are at work, during the night, when you are in and out of shops and your body is struggling to regulate temperature. Think about the last week, where and how many times did you have a hot flush?

Coping strategies

There are many practical coping strategies for hot flushes. I expect you already use a few – for example, many women benefit from using products like a cooling pillow, scarves or clothes. At work are you able to sit near a window, or leave a meeting, or are you comfortable riding it out. If so, how? Sometimes you may not be able to see how you can change things until you take a step back – and then it may seem obvious. Think about all the resources you already have, focus on the ones that work best and write them down.

Known triggers for hot flushes

Circle the triggers below that may worsen your hot flushes? These are common ones, but you may want to add your own. Some are within your control to change and some may not be, but you can find ways to manage them.

- Spicy food
- Coffee or alcohol
- Wearing warm clothes
- Change of temperature
- Smoking
- Stress
- Obesity
- Some health conditions
- Location

Cooling down your flush

At home

In the workplace

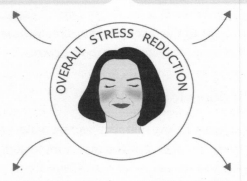
OVERALL STRESS REDUCTION

In the bedroom

Other

Now use this image to think about the adjustments you can make in a particular environment that will help you to manage and reduce hot flushes. You can download a copy of this worksheet from www.penguin.co.uk/mindfulmenopause.

Hypnosis and mindfulness support

Reducing stress will reduce the likelihood of having hot flushes. Taking steps to reduce stress is about creating a daily activity that helps you to manage it. For example, a sitting meditation in the morning can bring calm into your day, or a guided meditation just before you go to sleep can help to empty your mind of things that are troubling and worrying you. Other aspects of daily self-care can help such as exercise, crafting or reading. You can use the hypnotic Letting Go or download the Yoga Nidra meditation (see page 221), which is more of a mindfulness-based approach to reduce stress.

Where you are when you have a hot flush may increase your anxiety. At work, you may be concerned that your colleagues will notice, or if you have one at night you may worry about sleep disruption making you fatigued the next day. Learning how to reverse that and switch from anxiety into calm the moment the hot flush begins, can help you to reduce the severity of it. Anxiety without hot flushes can make you feel hot and bothered, so reducing anxiety in general and in the moment is about switching on your cooling system.

Using breathing techniques, you can learn to turn your awareness towards the rising sensation in your body. When you are present and calm, you are supporting your soothing system – you can also call this your cooling system. Allow the flush to move through.

'When I slow my breathing down, I activate my cooling system.'

Tip: Use your Calm Breath (see page 45).

EXERCISE 55: HEAT WAVES, COOL THOUGHTS

This simple mindfulness exercise in which you notice and are curious about the hot flush can help to change your experience of it. It's coming, there is nothing you can do to stop it, so instead turn towards it and start to familiarise yourself with it. Be curious about it. Can you notice where it is and where it is not in your body?

As a hot flush starts to rise from within, take a deep breath and notice where it is rising from. Take a deep breath and notice how your body responds. Now switch your breath into a Calm Breath (see page 45), making sure that your out-breath is longer than your in-breath.

Keep noticing, keep breathing. If your armpits are sweaty, just notice that; if your back is sweaty, just notice it. In this moment you can't stop it, but you can allow it to pass through. If an anxious feeling arises, keep a cool head and use a positive suggestion such as, 'As I breathe in, I relax, as I breathe out I let it go.'

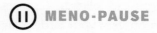 **MENO-PAUSE**

Hypnosis visualisations are also really powerful and are often a part of research studies. In the same way that imagining you are on a hot beach might help when you're cold, soothing and cooling imagery can help you to chill in the moment. While mindfulness is about awareness and acceptance, hypnosis is about awareness and change.

All you need to do is tap into your powerful imagination. I'm going to give you an example in the exercise below, but you can tailor this technique so it's very specific to you. The image doesn't have to be a snowy day; it can be a bucket of ice that you put your hand in or jumping into an ice-cold plunge pool or sitting on a giant ice cube. The possibilities are endless. When you imagine this 'cold' spot, the part of your brain that would experience it is activated sending a message to the body that you are cooling down.

❧ EXERCISE 56: TURNING DOWN THE HEAT

As a hot flush comes on fast, you need a hypnosis shortcut to switch you into a cool state within seconds. Conditioning it beforehand means that you can embed a word that will trigger that feeling of coolness really quickly, like a muscle memory in your brain. Then if you imagine being in your cool spot over and over again, you will build up a strong association of being cool with your word.

1. You can do this on your own or you can use the download (see page 9). All you need to do is find somewhere comfortable and close your eyes, using your Hypnosis Cloud and your deepener 10 . . . 1, to take you into the comfortable place of light hypnosis.
2. Then imagine it's a really cold day. You know those days in the middle of winter, when your breath is like a ripple of air that you can see floating on an icy

breeze. There is snow and ice, maybe deep snow or a very cold hoar frost. It's early in the morning and there is the muffled sound of the wind, and the branches weighted with snow or ice.

3. Really notice the details of the cold morning on your skin as you breathe in. I invite you to take your boots off, or your mittens, and plunge your feet or your hand into the snow. It's freezing, so cold, and that cold begins to move up through your foot or your hand like a silvery light. As it moves into your body, your body cools, the silvery cool light moving through every part of your body.

4. Now think of a word that you can connect to this experience. It might be cool, it may be silver, it may even be the place that you are imagining. It's up to you.

5. When you are feeling really cool, imagine that word in your mind.

Each time you repeat this visualisation using this word, you create a stronger association between the word and being able to introduce a cooling sensation into your body.

Tip: You can also use your Control Room (see page 53) for this and have a 'flush dial'. Imagine turning that dial down during a flush.

Reframing

Hot flushes are seen differently across different cultures; some see them as the rising of wisdom, the unlocking of a deeper knowledge and power that is granted to you as you move into your next life chapter. Like any other rite of passage, physical experiences can sometimes take you to the edge of what you think you are capable of, but when you learn how to be open to the power of change in your body, and to work with it, you invite your mind to witness your strength and resilience. As that energy rises up through your body, can you imagine your hot flushes as your Wisdom Waves? Or you may prefer the term power surge, one that is commonly used.

EXERCISE 57: COOLING BREATH

This very simple breathing exercise cools down the body. If you have a tongue that curls, use that to draw the air in; if you don't, imagine that you are sucking in the air like a straw. Breathe in through your tongue or imagine breathing in like sucking through a straw. Then put your tongue on the roof of your mouth and breathe out slowly through your mouth.

Repeat this five times or more if you need.

Summary

If you experience flushes – not all women do – start to notice whether there is a pattern associated with anxiety or stress. Stepping out of the spiral of anxiety can start to reduce their impact and improve your experience. Take a more introspective approach and recognise that hot flushes are not separate from you, they are part of you. Use the tools in this chapter to connect with and observe what is happening in your body. Be curious about your flushes, allow them to move through you and make practical adjustments that help you to feel more comfortable.

12

Getting Off the Anxiety Train

Anxiety is the dizziness of freedom.

Søren Kierkegaard

Whether it was when you were starting a new job, taking part in a sports event, or even your first day at school, most people will agree that they have felt anxiety at some point in their life. During perimenopause even those who haven't, or don't consider themselves as anxious, can be knocked sideways by unexpected anxiety.

How anxiety manifests can feel a little different for everyone; it can take the form of social anxiety, discomfort in places where you may have felt comfortable before, or a sudden rush of heightened awareness. You might have been a traveller, able to throw a few things into a backpack and just go, but now find that you aren't as spontaneous as you used to be. This is a common type of anxiety around menopause, and beyond.

'I notice the feelings of anxiety as
they rise, take a deep breath and I
let them gently go as they subside.'

These feelings can stop people doing the things that they love, and that they want to do. The clients I see don't want to stop going to visit family or going on adventurous holidays, but they feel as if they are unable to because of the intense feelings that they are having. I see this emerge so much with women from the ages of around 45–60; it's as if everything is felt more intensely. In this chapter we'll explore these feelings of anxiety in more depth.

Is it just menopause?

Often when women reach their mid-40s onwards, perimenopause becomes the scapegoat for all anxiety when in fact the source of it may be something completely different. A problematic relationship in the workplace, concerns about children or parents, an empty nest, a difficult marriage or partnership, feeling overwhelmed by life in general – all these, and more, can trigger anxiety. Hormonal fluctuations may heighten anxiety that already exists, but may not be the root cause – as much as we are led to believe they are responsible for everything!.

Learning what triggers your anxiety can help you disentangle the everyday anxiety from hormonally charged waves of anxiety. It's true that if you are already feeling anxious about anything else at home or work, menopause can throw a spotlight on it and give it a bit more charge, but if you are willing to address or find ways of managing the underlying trigger, the anxiety can crumble away.

Listen to your feelings

Sometimes feelings are a way of your body and mind trying to tell you something. I invite you to start thinking of anxiety in this way. Instead of trying to get rid of it, you start to meet it and wonder what it is trying to tell you. You can use the Name It To Tame It exercise on page 21 to help you explore these feelings.

'When I was 55, suddenly I was unable to sit in a music recital or a theatre, though I loved going. Through the work I did with my therapist I learned that the anxiety was triggered by a memory of my father's funeral. As I sat at the front in the middle, I yearned to get out and run away but I couldn't. I hadn't made the connection, but my anxiety was the grief I had felt in this moment. I was reminded of it each time I sat at an event. I started by noticing and acknowledging my grief, then accepting the feeling for what it was. With some hypnosis I was able to start sitting on the end of a row at the back and slowly I was able to enjoy going to the theatre again.'

Melanie

EXERCISE 58: WHAT'S STOPPING YOU?

Next time you have an event coming up that is creating anxiety for you, stop, take a deep breath and notice the feeling.

1. **What do you want to do?** Think about what you want to do – it may be going to the theatre, on holiday, even shopping. It could be a new experience, or it could be something that you have regularly done for many years and suddenly found harder to do.

2. **How much do you want to do it?** Use a scale of 1–10, with 10 being 'I really want to do this' and 1 being 'I absolutely don't want to do this.'

3. **Name three reasons why you wish to do it.** These are the reasons why you want to do it, not why you should do it! This is something for you, not your friends, your partner, your children, or anyone else.

4. **How happy would you be if you missed it?** First think about how happy you would be on a scale of 1–10 if you missed it, with 10 being the happiest?

5. **What do you need to know in order to feel safe and secure?** Think about why you are anxious. It may be fear of missing the train or plane, or sitting in the middle of a row and not being able to get out when you need to. You may not even know why you are anxious – if you don't, you can do the visualisation below and stop and start it when you notice anxiety rising. It's a great way of breaking down an anxiety into manageable chunks and identifying where it is coming from.

6. **What needs to be in place for you to enjoy it?** Think of all the things that need to change in order for you to feel safe, comfortable and free of anxiety. It may be catching an earlier train or getting a taxi

home. It may be the time of day, the amount of luggage you are carrying, who you are with, the food you will eat. What adjustments can you make so that it becomes easier for you?

Now, once all those adjustments are in place, close your eyes, use your Hypnosis Cloud (see page 49) and play it like a film, with you watching it. Notice how much any anxiety reduces or even disappears altogether.

If for any reason it doesn't, think about what needs to change in that image and go back to the last two questions. What do you need in order to feel safe, and what needs to be in place so that you can enjoy it?

You have a remote control to fast-forward and rewind when you need. Keep directing – adjusting and altering the film until it's finished and you are completely happy with it.

Then imagine stepping into the beginning of the film and press play. If you feel anxious at all, stop the film with your remote control, imagine yourself floating out of it, and then make the adjustment, until the anxiety is gone.

The more you practise this, the easier it becomes – it's amazing how quickly this works once you are familiar with the process.

If you scored highly on number 4 and are very happy to miss it, then question your motivation to go. If you are going because someone else wants to go, and it's not something that you would really want to do even if you were free of anxiety, ask yourself, 'Can I say no?'

A medical cause?

It's not just women that put all anxiety down to hormonal fluctuations – some doctors do, too. This is often at the expense of spotting a real physiological problem. There are several medical conditions that can contribute to anxiety, and it's important to rule these out. Conditions such as hyperthyroidism, anaemia, fibromyalgia and systemic lupus can cause anxiety and depression, but are often missed and put down to perimenopause. Consider speaking to your doctor about looking more closely at what you are experiencing. Sometimes we intuitively know when something isn't right, so if your little voice is speaking up listen to it and persist!

'It's easier for me to say things out loud, rather than internalising, "I'm feeling really cross this week." I've always been a really positive person, so it's hard for my friends. They don't expect to hear about anxiety or anything negative from me. The secret for me in getting through this stage is learning to live with a certain amount of uncertainty.'

Sara

Knowing the signs

It's helpful to recognise what signs your body is giving you, so you can begin to turn those moments of anxiety around and ground yourself using the technique on page 58.

When you stop to notice a difficult feeling rising within you, you can choose to give that feeling space to make its voice heard – to recognise and name it can be a way to learn more about yourself.

Mind

You may experience these thoughts and feelings as:

- Mood swings
- Worrying about immediate family and the world around you
- Not wanting to be with other people, even if you have been very sociable before
- Sudden unexplained fears or phobias
- Feelings of helplessness
- Feeling as if everyone else is managing this better than you

Body

This physical experience of these may be:

- Shortness of breath
- Butterflies in your stomach
- Heart palpitations
- Brain fog

Anxiety can feel incredibly isolating, but be reassured that you are not alone in this experience. There are many women who have sat in a chair across from me and said, 'But I should know how to manage this by now' or 'I used to be so adventurous and carefree, but now I feel anxious even going to the cinema.' Unable to shrug off daily worries with the same type of ease as they could when they were younger, the cumulative weight of them can become a heavy and tiresome burden to carry.

Sometimes it can feel as if your world is shrinking, and day-to-day life can be a struggle – you may start becoming anxious about anxiety itself. Lack of discussion around this exacerbates what is a very common and manageable experience of perimenopause. Thankfully, there are techniques you can learn to support your body and mind daily.

EXERCISE 59: LADDER BREATH

This breath can help you to climb out of an anxiety spiral – those moments when your breathing is getting faster or you are experiencing some of the signs in the above section. It's a very simple image to recall and keep in your mind, connecting you to a soothing rhythm that is similar to a grounding breath.

Use the image below to help you. Aim to slow your breath down so that each breath equates to a second.

Breathe in – 1 2 3 4 5 pause,
Breathe out – 5 4 3 2 1

Tip: It can be helpful to imagine this image in your mind as you do it.

Anxiety ladder

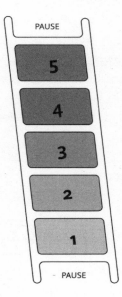

EXERCISE 60: TURNING ANXIETY AROUND

This is a very simple exercise for stopping anxiety in its tracks and the more you practise it, the easier it becomes.

- If you have a feeling of anxiety, notice where it is in your body. Imagine that it's a ball spinning around – notice which direction it is spinning in.
- Now imagine that ball has a colour and imagine holding your hands up to where the feeling is in your body. Your hands are like magnets and the ball starts to propel towards your hands.
- Imagine pulling that ball out of your body and into the air where it's suspended.

- Now you have control over that ball, start to spin it in a different direction to the current one – keep going. You may notice the anxious feeling is starting to subside.
- Now spin it in another direction and notice how it subsides even more.
- Keep spinning it until it disappears, or it takes off and floats away.
- Notice how much calmer you feel.

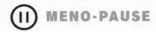 **MENO-PAUSE**

Become wise to anxiety

Persistently worrying or feeling on edge can manifest in a similar way to pre-menstrual experiences, otherwise known as pre-menstrual syndrome (PMS), something that you may have had throughout your life or only experienced temporarily. The hormonal fluctuations that you experience during your cycle are clearly defined as they are likely to have a pattern to them and even with irregular periods, you may still have been aware of PMS.

If you have had PMS in the past, you are more likely to experience similar symptoms during perimenopause; it's as if your body is more sensitive to hormonal adjustments. I know this might be difficult to hear, but at least by having knowledge of this, you know what to expect and understand what you are experiencing.

The difference is as your hormones wax and wane during perimenopause, these moments of anxiety and irritability can take you by surprise. However, you can learn how to recognise and manage them based on the experiences you have had with PMS.

What have you done in the past to reduce anxiety? Did you learn any tools? If yes, brilliant – you are off to a great start! Which tools have you used: yoga, meditation, relaxation exercises, having a nurturing bath?

EXERCISE 61: YOUR TOP FIVE ANXIETY BLASTERS

List five things that can get you out of a slump or a moment of anxiety – make sure that all five are free! Examples might be going for a walk, dancing, having a cup of tea, singing, snuggling up with a cosy blanket, crafting. If you wish, you can increase this to ten or more!

1. _____

2. _____

3. _____

4. _____

5. _____

Tip: When you are in a fog of anxiety, having mood-boosters to hand can make all the difference. Put these anxiety blasters in a positivity jar, so if you are having a tough day you can pick one out at random.

This next breathing technique is called alternate nostril breathing and when done regularly is an easy way to help your body and mind reduce anxiety. It brings balance to the sympathetic and parasympathetic nervous systems, as well as having additional benefits such as increasing focus and improving overall well-being.

EXERCISE 62: ALTERNATE NOSTRIL BREATHING

Look at the illustration to see where to place your thumb and fingers – your thumb is on your right nostril, your two middle fingers are between your eyebrows and your ring finger is just above your left nostril. Set yourself a timer for 3–5 minutes.

1. Take a deep breath in and out through both nostrils.
2. Then close your right nostril with your thumb.
3. Breathe deeply through your left nostril.
4. Cover your left nostril with your ring finger
5. Breathe out through your right nostril.
6. Inhale through your right nostril.
7. Cover up the right nostril and exhale through your left nostril.

Always finish on an exhale on the left nostril so you maintain a balance with both systems in your body. You can do this simple exercise as part of your morning or evening routine or just at those times when you feel anxious.

Unfinished business and trauma

Re-emerging trauma is something that can happen at this life stage. When I mentioned to a colleague that I was writing

Alternate nostril breathing

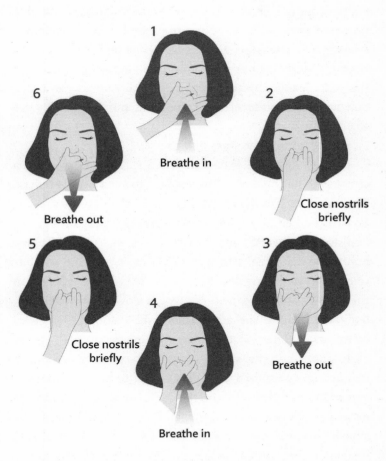

1. Breathe in
2. Close nostrils briefly
3. Breathe out
4. Breathe in
5. Close nostrils briefly
6. Breathe out

about it in this book, her response was 'Thank goodness!' She said, 'I see it all the time as well.' Recent research suggests that women who have experienced trauma in their lives are more likely to have stronger and more impactful experiences of menopause, particularly anxiety.

Enduring physiological symptoms of unresolved trauma are now better researched, and we know that trauma can disrupt hormonal systems in the brain and body that help it recover after stressful events. This means that at times when we are undergoing normal hormonal adjustments, such as in the years leading up to menopause, old traumas can break through and resurface, but sometimes not in the way we would expect.

Let me tell you the story of Inga . . .

My client Inga was in her late 50s. She had been away on a cruise with her husband. One evening the sea was turbulent. They went back to their cabin and her husband drew the curtains, as he had many times before. Suddenly Inga was terrified, and they had to keep the curtains open. When she came home, she didn't feel safe in small places; in fact, she was terrified of even getting in a car as a passenger. We worked on the feelings and the experience, and it slowly unravelled that her father, whom she adored and was wonderful in every other way, had disciplined her by shutting her away in a small dark space when she was very young. The physical feelings of fear and being trapped were very similar to the physical feelings of the turbulent sea, and the combination of that and the dark space were enough to trigger anxiety. We did some very simple trauma work to release that experience and to validate the experiences of feeling fear, but also of love for her father. In just a few sessions Inga's anxiety lifted completely.

As we grow through perimenopause, we are gifted opportunities to resolve previous trauma; it's as if our psyche knows that we have accumulated enough life experience, knowledge, wisdom and strength to resolve it. Lightening your load at this stage in your life can be liberating, and an invitation to confront powerful experiences that you may not have been able or ready to do before.

Imagine that every experience you have is dated, timed, labelled and filed away in the part of your brain that stores memories. When you experience a trauma, the brain doesn't file it away properly; it's like the to-do tray that's full to the brim with papers that need filing. If you do any trauma work, you can learn to file those memories where they are meant to be, not at the bottom of your in-tray where you are constantly reminded of them.

If you are perimenopausal and you can identify with this, it may be the perfect time to address and process previous trauma. There are many different approaches and I would strongly recommend finding someone who is experienced in trauma work.

Could this sudden onset anxiety be an invitation from your mind and body to resolve past trauma and to move forward into your next life stage? Can you find a way to recognise it as part of your life experience, but not as something that defines you in the present or your next life chapter?

Summary

If you find that you are more anxious or experiencing regular anxiety for the first time, learn to recognise your triggers. A daily practice of a sitting meditation, alternate nostril breathing, or listening to a guided hypnosis track on a regular basis can help reduce overall anxiety. On-the-spot techniques like the Ladder Breath and the Calm Breath are good for reducing anxiety if you are out and about.

13

The Last Taboo? Sex, Libido and the Menopause

I don't think the menopause in any way affects my sexual identity.

Nancy Friday

In nearly every book I have read and every study I've unpicked, menopause and sex seem to be a combination to be feared. It doesn't have to be this way. Sex and menopause is the last taboo, sometimes talked about with friends, but not always in detail. Instead, the internet often becomes the last recourse for women seeking an answer to what is happening to their sex drive and vagina.

Yes, your body will change, but your sex life doesn't have to be over; in fact, it can be the opposite. Sexual experiences can be liberating – an opportunity to connect more deeply with your body and with your partner.

Not all issues around sex at this life stage are because of menopause. You may be having less sex because of your relationship, or lack of relationship; it may because your partner isn't interested; it may be because you have children that might interrupt you or overhear; or you simply may not get any time alone. Being able to reflect on barriers to having sex can help you to identify where you may need a bit of support or to make changes.

You may slowly begin to realise that you are not as interested in sex. It can creep up on you – before you know it you haven't had sex for months, and have not really thought about it. This is more likely if your partner is experiencing a dip in their sex drive too.

Lack of awareness around this means that these shifts can take you by surprise. Our culture infrequently celebrates intimacy and rarely discusses sex among older people. Despite my hard work to normalise sex across the generations, my own teenage children are already conditioned to respond to anything in TV or literature as 'Eugh, old people sex' – I am considered 'old'.

With libido dropping and vaginal dryness that often causes pain, it can feel easier to just say, 'enough'. If you are anxious about having sex, it can cause a fight-or-flight response, which increases tension in the vagina – this can make sex more uncomfortable or it can manifest as vaginismus, where the vaginal muscles automatically tighten.

Tip: Use your Calm Breath (see page 45) before having sex, to relax your body and support your soothing system. Relax your hands and relax your jaw.

EXERCISE 63: SOFT AND OPEN

If you are finding that you are getting very tense before sex, you can use simple breathing exercises to calm your mind and body. Close your eyes and imagine a flower – maybe visualising a peony will relax you or a beautiful rose will be comforting. Picture a garden where you feel very relaxed.

Imagine the softness of the flower, perhaps early in the morning with dew on it. Notice it as the petals gently open, comfortably and easily.

Spend some time visualising this image three times a week or just before you have sex.

Tip: You can practise this visualisation by watching a time-lapse video of a flower unfurling. The more you watch it, the easier it will be to bring this powerful imagery to mind when you want to use it.

It can be easy to get stuck in a loop of not wanting to do anything about your sex life, because there is no drive to have it. It's no surprise that many women accept sex as something that they used to do.

Imagine a kettle of water heated over a fire. The water is always warm and can be heated up to boiling point quickly during your 20s and 30s, then as you go through your 40s that fire starts to dwindle, then perimenopause dampens it down or puts it out completely. You can get that fire started again, but it involves knowing how, then taking action to do that. Once you have what you need – matches, kindling and wood – you can start it up it and it can be as hot as it's always been.

You may be missing sex, not enjoying it, enjoying less of it or happy not having it at all. Finding the right balance within your own mind and within your relationship is something that may take some time, or it may not be an issue at all. Your body may be changing, which may knock your confidence or liberate you. Some women find great pleasure in deepening intimacy in different ways. It varies so much from person to person.

Surveys show that over 50 per cent of people over the age of 70 have an active sex life and some of those women are saying that sex is better than ever. It may be with their life partner, or a new partner. In a new world with more acceptance and diversity, there are women in their 40s and 50s who have been in heterosexual relationships all their life, suddenly finding themselves happy in a same-sex relationship.

Tantric sex

In Tantra, sex isn't just sex. It reaches beyond sex to explore the body, mind and spirit. A Tantric approach seeks to bring the body and mind into balance, opening opportunities to connect with powerful states of self-awareness. This approach is entirely compatible with this time in your life; it can shift the focus from performance to discovery, creativity and even spirituality.

And what about self-love! Women don't talk about masturbation much – another legacy of our culture. Masturbation doesn't have to replace sex with your partner, but in a time of transition it can give you the confidence and space to get to know your body intimately as it changes through the years of perimenopause and beyond. Self-exploration can help you build trust in your body. Connecting with your body both physically and emotionally and dropping into the feelings in your body on a regular basis through breathing, can help you to build a deeper energetic connection with it. You can learn to connect more deeply from your heart-space instead of sex being orgasm-centric.

> Masturbation is a meditation on self-love. So many of us are afflicted with self-loathing, bad body images, shame about our body functions, and confusion about sex and pleasure, I recommend an intense love affair with yourself.
>
> Betty Dodson

Whether you are on your own or with a partner, feelings may arise that are uncomfortable. They may be new, or they may have been there for years. Instead of avoiding or turning away from those feelings, you can start to learn about them and as you do that, you learn more about yourself and connect more deeply to sensations and feelings within you. This can be liberating as it can be an opportunity to release shameful or painful feelings relating to past experiences of sex.

You may find that you are less sensitive in some areas of your body and more sensitive in others. You may find that you are comfortable experimenting more with sex toys, either with or without your partner. There is so much that you can explore once you open yourself up to the opportunity of a new experience.

Sex doesn't have to stop – in fact, it can get better, but there are a few things you need to know to help you with that during perimenopause and in the years that follow.

Connection and communication

There are some wonderful online resources that discuss different aspects of women's experiences and give you encouragement as well as knowledge to ask the right questions. I've included these at the back of the book on page 11. Sometimes you will have to push for the support that you need. Being able to do that confidently is about being armed with information, realising that other women have done this – you are not in it alone – and knowing it can be different.

Tip: Use the BRAIN exercise on page 87 if you go to your doctor.

Your body will shift and change, you may find that sensitivity changes, and that you are having to relearn how your body responds. Opening up to your partner about your changing body and needs may be difficult, but it can make an enormous difference to your sex life. It may mean stepping into your own vulnerability, but if your partner's support matters to you then it's important. You can use the exercise on 174 to help you do this.

Are there friends that you can speak to honestly as well? Some may be more open to talking about sex than others. Alternatively, there are online forums where women discuss their sex lives anonymously.

Gratitude for your vagina

Your vagina is amazing. It expands and retracts just like a penis (have you ever heard the word atrophied penis?) and it may even have given birth – seriously, wow. Hopefully, it has given you lots of fun and pleasure over the years.

In some cultures, the vulva is worshipped, but in Western culture the historical medical phrase used to describe the vulva is Pudenda Membra, from the Latin meaning 'parts to be ashamed of'. The word vulva comes from the Latin meaning womb, so the word we use today still misrepresents our anatomy. This is the legacy we are currently dismantling.

As you grow older, in the years leading up to menopause, and those beyond, your vulva and your vagina may need a bit of TLC, along with other parts of you.

Learn about the products that can help you. Lubricants have been used for hundreds of years – according to historical records, olive oil was used going back to 350BC – and now there are also vaginal moisturisers, which can be applied on a daily basis. Look for natural products, try a few out and find what works for you. There is also oestrogen gel, applied vaginally, which is safe for women that cannot otherwise take oestrogen.

Sex and orgasm can help your vaginal muscles to stay toned, but there are also exercises that can help. Studies show that following a yoga programme with breathing and relaxation afterwards can improve desire, arousal, lubrication, orgasm and satisfaction, and reduce pain. Three out of four women in this study said that their sex lives had improved after following 12 weeks of daily yoga.

Atrophy is the awful word used to describe the vagina during the years around menopause. I think it should be banned from menopause language! Instead of seeing the words 'I have vaginal atrophy', in your mind I invite you to see 'I have a trophy vagina'. It's a typical hypnotic reframe, but this is about you owning your body and having gratitude for what it has done and what it can do in the future, with the right care, attention and love.

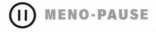 MENO-PAUSE

Above all, remember that your vagina is not the centre of everything when it comes to sex during perimenopause and beyond. Our view of sex rests within the limitations of a male paradigm – breasts, clitoris and vagina. Now is a time when you can move beyond this, if you haven't already.

Vaginal health

My focus is on helping you feel confident about your body, helping you to ask the questions you need to about your vaginal health – and keep asking those questions. If you have a drop in your libido and it's affecting you, speak to your doctor. If you have pain during sex, speak to your doctor. If you have ongoing Urinary Tract Infections (UTI), speak to your doctor. If there is general discomfort, speak to your doctor. Feeling able to ask questions means that you will get the support you need. Having the confidence to go back again and again is sometimes needed – you shouldn't be uncomfortable and in pain.

The fear of talking to a doctor is often rooted in shame about our bodies, and about sex. Some women also find it difficult to have intimate examinations because of a past sexual assault; if this is the case, then it may be helpful to see a talking therapist, or to speak to someone you feel comfortable with at your doctor's surgery or clinic to talk through what you are experiencing without having to have an examination.

You can learn to feel more confident about going to the doctor about your vaginal health. There are simple practical things that make a difference:

- Do your research beforehand and write your questions down so that you have something that you can refer to.
- Wear a long skirt, instead of having to take trousers off.

- Remember, you are always in control and can ask the doctor or nurse to stop at any time.
- Use your breathing exercises to relax beforehand.
- Ask for a female doctor.
- Ask for someone to accompany you, if that helps.

If your fear is stopping you from even making an appointment, use the following exercise to break it down.

EXERCISE 64: MAKING THAT APPOINTMENT!

Have two pieces of paper: on one write what your life will be like once you have got any help you need to make your day-to-day life the best it can be, free of any discomfort. On the other piece of paper write what your day-to-day life will be like if you don't get the support that could make such a difference.

- Now close your eyes and think of the first piece of paper, imagining what things would be like if those things were resolved and you spoke to someone who can give you the support you need. Bring up a vibrant colourful image, or a little film, in your mind of how you imagine your day-to-day life would be once these issues are resolved.

- Turn your attention to the other piece of paper and imagine your life if you didn't go to get the support you needed. Create that image or little film in black and white.

- Now bring up the colour image really big and bright, then switch it to the black and white one, then back to the colour one. The black and white one will start to become grey, and will disappear. Keep going until the black and white one is gone and you are left with the big colour image. You can then step into the colour image and become part of that experience, imagining what it's like once you have decided to get the support you need.

Pick up the phone and make that appointment!

Summary

A lot can be tied up in feelings around sex and intimacy. You may be more comfortable trying some of the things out in this chapter than others. Learn more about how you can explore your body. Seek help from a doctor or a talking therapist if you need to. Connect with your body through intimacy in a deeper way by using your breath, being curious about any feelings – emotional or physical, comfortable or uncomfortable.

14

Hair Loss

Someone once asked me 'How long does it take to
do your hair?' I said, 'I don't know, I'm never there'.

Dolly Parton

Hair is part of our lives and is woven into our culture. Young children often play with dolls, brushing their hair; perhaps you and your friend styled each other's hair – cementing a bond of close friends. Your mother or father may have brushed your hair every day – it may have been an unpleasant experience or a gentle loving connection. Your hair is often part of how people describe you – 'You know, the one with the short brown bob' or the 'Curly redhead'.

Lovers may have run their fingers through your hair, strangers may have commented on it, tried to touch it. You may have lost it through illness and watched it grow again, your identity re-establishing itself in your shifted world.

Your hair can have a huge impact on your identity and is an important part of who you are. We often define ourselves by our hair – the colour, the shape, the texture. We can hide behind our hair, creating personas with it. How we choose to wear our hair can be an expression of ethnicity, class, gender, religion and even of rebellion. It can be a loud statement or a way to blend in. But it's your hair, you know it and you recognise it. It's part of who you are.

Hair thinning

Hair thinning is one of the most devastating but lesser talked about aspects of menopause. If it is happening to you, I am so sorry. It's hard isn't it? I know because I experienced it in my early 40s. This aspect of menopause can be extremely distressing and despite feeling so burdened by it, women may feel it is vain to focus on and become stressed about this aspect of their looks. It isn't.

Hair is important – you will have had choice in how to wear your hair and may have used it as a way to express yourself. Hair salons are places that we go to regularly – they can be a place of community, a meeting of women, a place to gossip and chat. If you are losing your hair it can be a place to dread instead of something to look forward to.

Sexuality can also be connected with hair. In our culture it's often defined by fashion, and everywhere we look there are women showcased with lush, long tresses. It's a sign of youth and beauty. Losing hair is a sign of becoming older and the impact of it can take you by surprise.

Before hair loss, you could cover those stray whites with highlights and dye, having some control over how you presented yourself. Thinning hair is a whole new ball game and can make you question the very heart of who you are.

Hormones, nutrition or stress?

Research suggests that hair loss during menopause is because of a mix of hormones, ethnicity and genetics. Oestrogen, testosterone and progesterone help hair grow faster and stay on your head for longer. As those hormones drop, hair grows more slowly but also thins as it drops out sooner.

That little hair on your chin that has sprouted? That's also hormone related. It does seem a bizarre quirk of nature that the hair on our heads drops out, yet it's important to have them on our chin. You can only laugh at this and buy a good pair of tweezers.

Although hormones can influence hair changes, they are not the only reason why hair can thin or fall out. What you eat can also have an impact, so it's worth investigating dietary changes. You can use the tools in Chapter 15 to motivate yourself to make lifestyle changes around food. How you style your hair can also have an impact – traction alopecia from braids that have been tightly tied can be more pronounced during menopause, and heat treatments can weaken hair.

Hair loss can be associated with stress and in extreme cases, people can experience alopecia, when their hair drops out over a matter of days or weeks. Addressing stress can optimise hair growth by helping to balance your hormones. Taking steps to reduce stress by introducing daily habits of introspection or self-care is one of the best things that you can do when it comes to hair loss. Not only does it optimise the environment for growth, but it will help you become more resilient in the face of any hair loss.

It's not just the daily stress that you can learn to let go of; it's the stress of 'finding a cure' that is so persistent with hair loss. It is a billion-dollar industry and there are so many alleged cures, you can get lost in a cornucopia of snake oils. It can get expensive and it can sometimes feel as though a solution is a pipe dream, but people can still be seduced into thinking that there is one unique combination of treatments that will work for them. Sadly, I've found that pursuing this can create more stress.

'I found hair loss devastating. I can't begin to describe how it made me feel. It was as if I no longer identified with who I thought I was. The person looking back at me in the mirror wasn't someone I recognised. It was disconnecting on so many levels. I researched and researched shampoos, treatments, transplants, you name it. I spent a fortune trying to fix it, so I could once more recognise the person looking back at me in the mirror. Having found some evidence that rosemary oil could stimulate the scalp, I tracked down a rosemary tonic with good reviews and applied it diligently. It seemed to really work! At the same time I also worked on how I related to the loss, along with upping my meditation practice and self-care. I'll never know if it was the rosemary oil, or how I learned to care for the new person looking back at me, but my hair is now thicker – not the same as it once was, but I'm happy and that's all that matters really isn't it?'

Sophie

In truth one of the most effective treatments for preventing hair loss is to stop looking for treatments and to learn to redefine yourself. That way the stress drops away. You have everything within yourself, each and every day, to grow into your new style, your new way of being.

You are much more than the hair on your head.

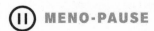 **MENO-PAUSE**

Be kind to your hair!

How do you speak to your hair? Do you use language like 'I hate my hair,' 'My hair is awful today,' 'My hair is misbehaving' or 'If you do that again, I'll tear my hair out'? Your hair is a part of you. How you speak to your hair is in part how you speak to yourself. Can you learn to speak to your hair kindly? It may be having a really tough time right now, it may be struggling a bit, it may need some compassion.

EXERCISE 65: COMPASSION CONDITIONER

Every day notice the hair that you have on your head. Really notice it, notice its colour, how it is that day, notice the thinner patches and the small hairs growing up. Just notice them and accept them. If you catch a feeling of loss or sadness coming up, name it and then let it go. Then come back to just noticing. Imagine that you are tenderly nurturing those hairs with love. Give your hair compliments and make it feel good about itself:

1. Good morning hair.
2. Thank you for being here today.

3. I love the way that (you are curling today, falling, your colour is).

4. How do you want to be worn today?

If your hair is falling out in the shower or on your brush, let it go and thank it for being a part of your life.

Be playful!

If you are finding the transition hard, then you may want to learn how to be playful. If you have never worn wigs, hats or hairpieces, then step inside the incredible colourful world of artificial hair!

Depending on your ethnicity or cultural background, this may be deeply rooted in your culture and nothing new to you, or you may be someone who is astounded to learn just how many women use hairpieces and wigs. As no one really talks about it and because they are so realistic nowadays, it is hard to tell if someone is wearing one! When a friend once whispered in my ear 'Google hair toppers', I went straight home and discovered an area of the internet I never knew existed. Use this as an opportunity for exploration – and, remember, ultimately a wig is just a hairy hat! You can experiment with headbands, find beautiful hats, learn how to wear a headscarf.

Choose to see this as a part of your menopause journey, your transition. Sometimes this means needing to explore this aspect of yourself in different ways and being curious about the attachment you have to your identity, before reaching a place of acceptance. You may find that you come full circle and ultimately feel liberated by not having to spend a lot of money and time on surface impressions and feel a comfortable sense of living with your own hair, an expression of you.

Wisdom white

How often do you open magazines and see women with white hair spread across a feature? Fortunately, more and more women are owning their white hair, and seeing the beauty in it. Yet, if you google white hair, some of the headings are 'White hair and how to prevent it', 'Combat white hair'.

Your white hair is quite literally your crowning glory! It's representative of your wisdom, your experience, your knowledge. The white hair that emerges from your head is nature's crown. Wear it with pride, you earned it.

White hair can be caused by hormonal changes and changes in the scalp as we age, but it can also be because of other influences in your life. Nutrition, your genes and stress are all part of changes to your hair colour during menopause. A recent study at Harvard University found that noradrenaline, a neurotransmitter produced by the brain in minor and chronic stress situations, seems to affect the pigment-producing skin cells that give your hair its colour. We know that shock can turn hair white overnight in extreme circumstances, but we know much less about how ongoing stress can do the same.

While you can always learn ways of managing stress, you will have met, and will continue to meet, challenges that trigger stress during your life, this is normal – these challenges and how you met them, overcame them, and what you learned from them have added to your knowledge base. Every hair on your head that is white is a symbol of what you have learned, the wisdom that resides within you.

'I wear my crown of white with
pride.'

Metamorphosis

One of my clients had been struggling with hair loss and had
been working on acceptance and gratitude around it. She told
me that one morning she had felt there was more hair falling
out than usual, so she had done a gratitude practice, thanking
the hair for its time in her life and let it go. As she sat in front of
the mirror, without any make-up, after drying her hair, which
was unbrushed, flyaway and white, she said that for the first
time it felt as if she was shedding a skin and that she was
emerging as a wild woman with white hair, her head held high
and heart open, free of expectations that had burdened her.
Rather than feeling despondent and dreading losing her hair,
in that moment she felt a sense of lightness, relief and
liberation.

Of all the aspects of perimenopause losing hair is one of
the most physical metaphors of metamorphosis. It *is* like the
shedding of a skin and a visible reminder of moving from one
life stage to the next.

EXERCISE 66: MIRROR IMAGE

Next time you sit in front of a mirror without your make-up,
with your hair untamed, don't just look at what isn't there,
or what is disappearing; instead look at what is appearing.
See the wild, wise woman in you. Her depths deeper than
the ocean, her heart fuller than the sky of stars, her eyes a

reflection of the universe. She is full of experience, strong and beautiful.

- Sit tall, with your shoulders back.
- Take a deep breath in and slowly breathe out.
- With your next breath in, notice your heart and breathe down as far as you can into your heart space, feeling a fullness of love.
- As you breathe out, imagine breathing love to the woman in front of you.
- Then imagine that love coming back to you with your next breath in.
- Feel the power and connection with the woman in front of you.
- Thank you for being you.

Summary

Hair loss can be more devastating on many levels than people want to admit. It's not just about vanity and it's okay to allow yourself to recognise that loss and grieve for that part of you. Remember to be kind and loving towards all those parts of your body, down to the tiniest hair on your head. Learn to love your metamorphosis, be playful with it. Whether you choose to embrace your new slimline hair or decide to have a go with enhancements is up to you. I encourage you to just have fun!

15

Letting Go of Weight, and Loving Well-being

The question is not what you look at,
but what you see.

Henry David Thoreau

Weight. It is one of the most common reasons why people come to see me, often after they have tried everything else. I learned a lot from this in the early years of my practice, and I discovered how important it is to begin to cultivate perimenopause-friendly habits around food and movement.

This can be the types of food you are eating, the type of exercise you do, and your attitude towards your changing body. Whichever stage you are at, there are simple tools that can help you to create a healthy mindset that supports your changing body. You will learn to create habits that motivate and encourage you, but also give you permission to let go of patterns that no longer serve you.

There is a huge amount written on weight, and weight-loss – it's a billion-dollar industry. And it's all about being slim. What does it mean to be slim? What is it going to bring you? How is it going to change things for you? You may be perfectly happy in the body you have right now, or you may want to make changes for well-being reasons.

My approach is focused on helping you understand your relationship to food, your body and your emotions. During perimenopause it becomes even more pertinent as we learn that our changing bodies need a different and kinder approach. You may have been working hard at the gym, running, eating less, without seeing any change. To see change, first your thinking has to change.

Menopause is a time to start:

- Tuning into your body's needs.
- Learning about how different types of foods can support this stage of your life.
- Moving in ways that support your hormones and your bones.
- Recognising the impact of thoughts and feelings on your body.

The practical tools in this section can build on any knowledge you've already learned around healthy eating and exercise by helping you to learn the language of your body. Because sometimes it feels as if it's speaking a different language, doesn't it?

Hypnosis for letting go of weight is about being healthy and feeling comfortable in your own skin.

Hormones: a weighty issue

Hormonal changes mean physical changes. Gaining weight is one of the first notable shifts in perimenopause, sometimes even casually referred to as 'baby weight that I'm still carrying' 'or the stubborn midriff'. How often do you hear, 'My metabolism has slowed down and now I'm gaining all this weight'?

It's true that as oestrogen drops, your metabolism slows down and this does affect your body – sadly, midlife metabolic changes do not take a love of cheese and cake into account. However, metabolism is not the only contributory factor to the midlife spread, and contrary to popular opinion, studies show that low oestrogen in itself does not cause weight gain. It may lead to an increase in total body fat, in particular abdominal fat, but weight gain, appetite and choice of foods are often influenced by other aspects of perimenopause such as lack of sleep.

Using scales is not my way as a therapist, though I accept that some people find weighing themselves regularly motivating – it's really up to you. If you feel deflated when standing on the scales, but feel good in what you are wearing, chuck the scales away – they are no measure of who you really are. An honest exploration of lifestyle and how you can make changes that support your whole system through meditation, mindfulness, visualisation and hypnotic suggestion is a sustainable and liberating way to gain new perspectives on your body. Letting go of weight means letting go in other ways.

'I allow change to happen in a gentle and loving way.'

How has your lifestyle changed?

As you move into your menopause years, you may not be running around young children as much, you may have a more sedentary job or have started to work part-time. You may not be going out as much (dancing on a night out can be a turbo-charged aerobic routine with added endorphins). Even small shifts like this can, over time, start to alter your body. There may be interruptions to your life that break a gym or walking routine. You may be taking on other family responsibilities that mean abandoning your own self-care.

'I feed my body healthy nourishing food because it deserves to be taken care of.'

Think about the last ten years and write down in your journal small changes that may have led to a more sedentary lifestyle. It's helpful to understand the bigger picture so that you can start to integrate new habits into your day that keep you moving and energised.

The impact of anxiety and stress

Anxiety and stress can have an impact on weight and physical well-being because of the decrease in progesterone and oestrogen that you learned about in Chapter 3. Fluctuations in weight can be linked to anxiety and stress, because of spikes in the stress hormone cortisol.

From an evolutionary perspective, if you are in fight-or-flight mode (see page 118), or stressed, your body will crave energy foods, because you need fast, high energy to fight and run away. Weight gain related to stress tends to be around the middle of your body.

Cortisol is naturally higher during menopause, and so it really pays to proactively find ways to empty your daily stress and support your soothing system.

A daily meditation practice and some hypnosis guided meditations to let go of stress will support any intention to live and eat in an intuitive and connected way – listening deeply to the needs of your body, rather than relying on the familiar quick fixes.

Why a healthy weight matters

My approach is always to be reassuring and encouraging, realistic and positive. I'm not telling you anything that you don't know. It's common knowledge that excess weight can exacerbate some aspects of menopause. When my friends often casually mention that their hot flushes have started up again, I usually ask, 'Is there anything stressful in your life, or have you gained some weight?'

If you are still thinking in terms of BMI as a guide, stop! This is effective less than 50 per cent of the time when measuring obesity and takes no account of different ethnicities or women that are perimenopausal!

Nowadays personal trainers encourage people to measure rather than weigh. It's up to you to think about what motivates you, and to create the habit of being motivated to do what you know is right for you.

Even though you may think you don't understand what your body is doing right now, and why it's not doing what it used to do, you still know it better than anyone else and you can learn to tune in to what it needs. It may take some perseverance and patience, as well as trying new things out. When a client comes to see me about weight issues, usually they already know what they need to do – our work together is about finding the blocks to achieving those goals and feeling good about themselves.

Nutrition, gut health and the menopause

by Jenny Tschiesche BSc (Hons) Dip (ION) FdSc BANT

The health and function of your whole digestive tract (known as your 'gut health') can be affected by the hormonal changes that occur prior to, and during the menopause. Levels of the stress hormone cortisol and the sex hormone oestrogen change during this period and it is this change that leads to poorer gut health. Cortisol increases in the time leading up to menopause, levels get even higher during the menopause. Not only is cortisol linked to stress but a high level over a longer period is also linked to depression.

Eating behaviours during times of stress and depression mean that some people eat a lot more, especially processed and sugary foods, while others go the other way, consuming almost nothing. Both can be detrimental to gut health and lead to a poor relationship with food that can exacerbate stress and depression.

High levels of cortisol can lead directly to gut issues too, ranging from indigestion, low stomach acid, poor digestive enzyme production, to problems including small intestinal bacterial overgrowth (**SIBO**) and increased intestinal permeability. Common symptoms of these conditions include food intolerance, gas, wind, bloating, cramping and constipation.

While there are behaviours that make gut health worse during this period, there are many positive and preventative actions that you can take to try and mitigate against poor gut health. These focus on improving the health and integrity of the gut lining, rebalancing the bacteria in the gut and improving hormonal balance.

Don't	Do
Eat mindlessly	Eat mindfully
Forget to drink water	Drink sufficient water
Crash diet	Eat more greens
Eat fast food	Focus on prebiotic foods
Skip meals	Get sufficient exercise
Drink too much caffeine	Sleep enough
Eat sugary foods	Eat fermented foods
Leave stress unaddressed	Enjoy good fats

The language of weight

A good hypnotherapist will not talk about 'losing weight'. What is your unconscious desire if you lose something? Usually, it's to find it again! Instead of losing weight, think about letting the weight go, or finding your healthy balance.

'I feel so much lighter when I let weight go.'

This use of language around weight is also recognisable in words like 'fulfilled'. The brain works in a very literal way; if you are not fulfilled in life, you may choose to be full-filled in other ways. Other common themes are the use of food to literally push feelings down. Not feeling 'satisfied' in your life can lead to other ways of meeting the need for satisfaction.

If you are stressed or agitated and restless, you may not even be aware of the uncomfortable feeling arising, the fridge door opening, the hand reaching inside, and the food that you are chewing. With mindfulness you can learn to connect with that feeling, instead of pushing it down, learn about it and let it go. Meeting the feelings rather than pushing them away creates an opportunity to let them go.

Sometimes feelings and attitudes around food go right back to your childhood and have been established as uncon-scious patterns over the years. Were you told to 'finish all the food on your plate'? Did you go hungry or have to be quick to battle siblings for food? Was there a relative who baked for you, or cooked for you with so much thought that it made you feel cared and loved? Unbeknownst to us those patterns are well and truly rooted in our belief system, driving our behav-iours around food.

If you recognise this in yourself, midlife can be a great time to start to acknowledge those behaviours and patterns. As you go through menopause and beyond, unfinished business tends to surface, so you can put it to bed and feel free to explore your life on your terms, feeling comfortable in your own skin.

EXERCISE 67: THE STOP SIGN

This exercise is a mix of mindfulness and hypnosis. When behaviours are unconscious, like snacking, hypnosis can give you a big reminder to STOP! Then awareness of the feeling can emerge, helping you to learn to notice the feeling that comes up at that time. In my experience a combination of the two creates more lasting changes.

Step 1: Hypnosis. Imagine a time when you are snacking, opening the fridge, eating something that you know you'll regret afterwards. Close your eyes and connect with that feeling. When you connect with it, imagine a giant red stop sign popping up in front of you with lots of Klaxon alarms going off around you, like a noisy sports game. Repeat this three times every day for a week.

Step 2: Mindfulness. When you go to snack, the stop sign will flash up, reminding you to stop and connect with the feeling that is driving the snacking.

- Take a deep breath, and connect with that feeling.

- Where is it in your body? Just notice it.

- Name the feeling – boredom, stress, anxiety, thirst, hunger?

- Just notice it with loving kindness and let your heart smile at it.

Tip: You can then learn to meet the need that has emerged in a different and healthier way. If you are stressed, can you do a guided meditation before you go to sleep? If you are bored, can you do something that stimulates you?

Wake up willpower!

There are two aspects of your brain when it comes to desire: the first is your hot head, which is an impulsive part that wants things 'now!' The second is your cool head – calm and collected, this part is focused on what you really want long term.

When you want to make long-term adjustments, there is often conflict between these two parts. The hot-tempered part is driven by emotion and feeling, while the cool-headed part is clear about the path you need to take to succeed in the goals you have set.

Sometimes when the hot head thinks it is easier to just sit on the sofa and watch TV, the cool head is the part of you that says, 'Hey, remember your goal to get on top of this meno-pause game? Come on, you're going to feel great when you get up and go for a walk.' Your cool head is skilled at making you do the 'harder thing'.

Mindfulness and hypnosis can help to support your cool head, which is your pre-frontal cortex. It's like a muscle – the more you exercise it, the stronger it gets.

Temptations challenge the hot head, activating the reward centre of your brain and releasing dopamine – this flood of dopamine amplifies any 'in the moment desires', leaving you less concerned about long-term goals. It hard for the cool head to make its voice heard in these circumstances. Next time you see temptations at the checkout in a shop, be alert to the marketeers' tricks . . . they know how to activate your hot head and they make plenty of money out of it!

In perimenopause there are changes to your pre-frontal cortex that may make it harder for your cool head to always do its job. This is why mindfulness is so beneficial – it helps maintain and even grow grey matter in this part of your brain. Self-compassion has been shown to contribute to greater motivation and self-control – it strengthens willpower. Being kind to yourself and letting guilt go, or even better, not feeling guilty at all, means that you are more likely to meet the goals that you are setting yourself.

'I let guilt go and am comfortable with my choices.'

You can support your cool head by moving! There is a growing body of research that suggests exercise helps to strengthen your pre-frontal cortex. A great activity for menopause is an 'awe walk' as it has a multitude of benefits. A recent study showed that older adults who took 15-minute daily walks over a period of eight weeks, showed positive emotions and less stress, activating their soothing system. Awe is the sense of something larger than yourself, something that perhaps you cannot fully understand – for example walks in nature, music, a protest march, even visiting an ancient built environment that inspires awe. Both collective as well as solitary experiences can trigger the positive emotion of awe.

EXERCISE 68: A MINDFUL AWE WALK

Walking is a great form of exercise to do during menopause and beyond. It's good for bone strength and mental well-being. You can boost an awe walk by doing the walk mindfully. To do this find somewhere that meets the awe criteria, somewhere that you get a sense of the world being bigger than yourself and that creates a sense of marvel.

Awe can be of a mountain or it can be the formation of the bark on a tree. Or it can be a small woods or park near where you live.

1. Ground yourself before you start. Notice your feet on the ground, and take a deep breath all the way up through your body from the soles of your feet to the top of your head. Connect with your breath (see page 44), in through your nose and out through your mouth, connecting with the earth beneath your feet and the sky above you.

2. Now turn your attention to the sounds around you – just notice them. Breathe in deeply and breathe out.

3. Turn your attention to the vastness of your surroundings, what brings awe. Notice it. Breathe in and breathe out.

4. Turn your attention to what's in your vicinity – it may be a leaf, moss, an insect. Notice the details in it, the way it moves, the way it feels underfoot, the way it smells or the way it feels. Breathe in and breathe out.

Keep walking, keep noticing, keep breathing. You don't have to walk far – you can walk slowly over a short distance.

Tip: If you take a long awe walk, you can walk briskly, punctuating it with mindful pauses to notice where you are, following the steps above.

Strengthening your pre-frontal cortex is something that meditation and mindfulness are known to help with. Your morning meditation, daily moments of mindfulness, awe walks and observations all start to strengthen your willpower and motivation.

You can learn to activate your willpower by recognising the battle going on between your hot head and your cool head – these are those moments when you really want to indulge in something, and you know that it's not in your plan. In these moments get into your cool head by using your Calm Breath (see page 45), then use the Name It To Tame It exercise on page 21. This will help you to trigger your soothing system, which supports the willpower part of your brain, your pre-frontal cortex.

Tip: To add some self-hypnosis, visualise your long-term goal when you are doing this.

EXERCISE 69: DETONATING MIND BLOCKS

If blocks come up time and time again, you can use hypnosis tools to clear them. A block can be an excuse or a feeling.

1. If you are coming to a block, imagine that block as a huge wall in front of you that is impossible to pass. The concrete or brick in that wall is made up of everything that is stopping you from achieving your goal.
2. Now imagine you have a pack of explosives. Place them all around the imaginary wall.
3. When you are done, at a safe distance get your charge set, pull the handle up and then when you are ready take a deep breath and focus on your goal, really focus on it.
4. Now bring the wall into your mind's eye again and then press the charge down, blowing up the block.

5. As the dust clears you can see light coming through, and a path ahead. Step through and continue on your path.

Tip: This visualisation can be used daily if you are struggling to meet your goal.

> 'Just for today I can [fill in the step you need to make].'

Making habits stick

If you have been yo-yo dieting all your life and are finding it difficult to establish a long-term change, get support. There are coaches, therapists and personal trainers that specialise in menopause. Find what works for you.

If you recognise that you are eating for emotional reasons, there are ways to change your response. Often the emotional drive for food is your mind seeking safety and security, albeit in an unconventional way. As well as being necessary for physical survival, food is also about emotional survival – as a human you need food to survive, and, depending on which culture you are from, food can represent love, friendship and community. All of which you may need more than ever during times of transition.

It's okay to have cravings; they can give you messages and insight. Instead of pushing the feeling away, connect with it and bring it into your awareness. Then you can work with it. Be curious about it – what is it telling you? Are you thirsty? Maybe have a glass of water – hunger and thirst messages can get confused sometimes. What do you need in this moment? It may not be food. Is this food going to make you feel better after you've eaten it? Try this simple exercise.

EXERCISE 70: TURNING THOSE CRAVINGS DOWN

This is a great exercise for a general or very specific craving, as it helps you identify the feeling and switch it off. I've had wonderful success with this and it's so easy to do.

- Next time you find yourself roaming the kitchen looking for food or you are battling a craving, stop and use your Calm Breath (see page 45) three times or ground yourself.
- Next turn your attention to the craving. Where is it in your body? Just notice it.
- If that craving had a sound, what would it be? Turn the craving into the sound.
- Now imagine a dial that controls that sound.
- Turn the sound right down until it has disappeared completely and for good.
- Notice how that feeling has disappeared.

'I successfully "turned down" my chocolate addiction, which has always been terrible. It definitely escalated during a difficult time and has been seriously hampering my ability to get into shape. However, I've just realised that in the last two weeks I've eaten all of two squares of dark chocolate a day and had no further desire for it. It's like a miracle, wow! Seriously can't believe it!'

Cat

By stopping and checking in with cravings, and food that you are choosing to moderate, you can start to understand the unconscious patterns.

🎧 EXERCISE 71: INTUITIVE EATING

This guided meditation will help you to support your intention to eat foods that your body needs to stay balanced, fit and healthy during this time of your life. You'll start to notice when you are full, when you are hungry, when you are thirsty. You'll find that you are automatically drawn to foods that support your body during menopause.

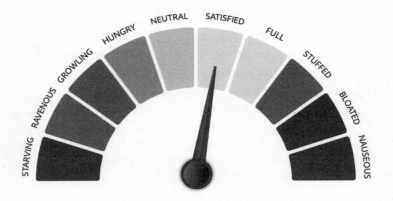

Intuitive eating

The Hunger Scale

You can listen to the meditation before you go to sleep at night or anytime that feel you need a boost.

Tip: Listen to it the night before you go for your weekly shop – you may find that your trolley is a lot lighter!

Tip: If you are craving something, can you wait ten minutes to see if the craving passes? Creating a habit of delayed gratification is shown to help train the brain to recognise and work out what you really need instead of what you want in the moment.

Carbohydrate cravings can mean you are fatigued. If you are having issues with sleep, as is common in menopause, you may be feeling the urge to eat more sugar and energy-rich food.

Learning to understand what your body is doing can give you the chance to make interventions that change how you meet your needs.

Small adjustments, big changes

In this section I want you to really get into the what and the why. Noticing the small adjustments that you can make on a daily basis can bring big changes to your life.

- Which foods do you crave?
- Which foods that you crave aren't fuelling your well-being?

They may be savoury or sweet.

Do you have associations with foods, people or places? If so who? Think about foods you love and would eat seconds of, even if you are not hungry. Think of the places that you have

eaten these foods and people who cooked and served something similar to you in the past.

> *'Spaghetti Bolognese is the best – I will always eat bowl-
> fuls of it given half a chance. Every Saturday growing up
> we would have bolognese made by my mother . . . and
> when we visited my grandparents overseas, whom I
> loved deeply, it was the meal I always looked forward to.
> It seems silly but it's a memory of my childhood before
> my father left my mother, and everything was happy.
> Now I'm writing this, all I am craving is bolognese, but I
> know that I am actually craving my family and the
> warmth of my grandmother's kitchen.'*

Alison

EXERCISE 72: NOTICING PATTERNS

Let's go into this a little deeper. When you start to think
about your response to food, and write it down, you may
start to see a pattern forming.

- Are there certain times of the day you eat more?

- Are there certain times of the day that you feel hun-
  grier, snack more or get cravings? Spend a few days
  just noticing what your body is telling you.

- Write down the times of the day you feel hungry and
  what you are craving.

_____

_____

Are there places you eat more? At home or at work, out with friends, in the car? Think about the places you snack: it may be at a desk, or in front of the TV, at a particular friend's house – why might that be? Are you afraid of saying no to the cakes your colleagues bring in? Do you have a friend that is a 'feeder'? It's okay to say I'm learning to say no. Sometimes other aspects of your personality and other people's personalities can derail the best-laid plans.

_____

_____

_____

Now reflect back on those lists and start to know those moments in your life, and those parts of you that are guiding your choices around food. Can you make at least three changes which you know will make a big difference?

_____

_____

_____

Now can you can start to see the bigger picture and make small adjustments and changes in a targeted way? Use the tools in this chapter to reduce craving, understand

associations and challenge yourself to do something different where you are making choices you would rather not
make.

Tip: Be creative. Instead of snacking, can you do something
else for ten seconds? Perhaps, run on the spot, shake it off
or use the Spotlight Technique on page 111.

Amelia came to me because she was eating unhealthy
snacks in the car. She'd stop for petrol and would fill up the
glovebox along with the fuel tank. Being in the car was the only
time she had space to really think uninterrupted – the stress of
work, home and other things in her life that were difficult were
pushed down with crisps and chocolate. She found the Name
It To tame It mindfulness exercise (see page 121) very helpful in
meeting those feelings, but she also discovered a love of podcasts in that space. With some hypnotic suggestion that every
time she got in her car 'she was successfully driving towards
her goal', it worked a treat.

Unconscious influences on weight

Sometimes it may be more complex than just changing patterns.
This is about how you feel at a deeply unconscious level. Sometimes the reason weight is hard to let go of is because a part of
you believes it protects you from danger. Bear with me! Trauma
without resolution can be a cause of weight gain. Your mind has
curious ways of keeping you safe from the world and learning to
understand it in this way may be the key that unlocks your story.
This is especially true for those women who have experienced
unwanted attention or sexual assault; it can be a way of making
someone feel safe by making themselves feel less visible.

A well-known hypnotherapist, David Elman, from around the 1950s, talked about a woman who'd had a fibroids operation. Afterwards, she had had a discussion with the doctor about whether the fibroids were malignant. The doctor said, 'Well you haven't lost any weight recently have you?' At the time the woman had been trying to lose a few pounds. When the doctor said this to her, she wasn't sure whether she had lost the weight because she'd been dieting or because of a malignant tumour. The suggestion stuck and she started to overeat as the unconscious thought was 'If I gain weight, then I don't have a tumour'.

Another case he describes is a woman who couldn't lose the 80lb she needed to have surgery – her response in hypnosis was 'I don't want to lose the other 80lb because then I'll be able to have surgery and I'm terrified of that.'

If this small section speaks to you, I'm sorry that you have had this experience. Even if you have seen a trauma therapist there is the option of seeing a counsellor or a therapist who specialises in your thoughts around weight. There is always the 'me you cannot see' – working with someone else can help you to learn about those parts of you in a positive and supportive way.

Mindful eating

I've given you lots of hypnosis tools – it's now time for some mindfulness-based interventions, which I love for menopause. Let's start with mindful eating, which is the act of being consciously aware of the connection between your body and the food you are eating. Unlike hypnosis, which is very goal-driven in terms of well-being and weight, mindful eating is not focused on diet, but awareness of what you are eating and the response your body has to that food.

When you eat consciously, you aim to turn your attention to the food you are eating. As well as the food itself, you can even be aware of its journey to your plate. The ingredients for your meal or the food you are eating may have been in the ground, watered by the rain and warmed by the sun. Someone may have picked them, then packed them, and cooked them. The meal itself shows your interconnection with the world around you and within you.

The attention you place on preparing and eating the food on your plate is not about diet or losing weight, it's simply about becoming acquainted with your body – its experience of hunger and its experience of being sated. When you become consciously aware of what you are eating and how you are experiencing it, you learn to respond to the relationship between the food on your plate and the feedback in your body. This way you can cultivate a more intuitive approach to eating what your body needs, not what your mind wants.

EXERCISE 73: EATING MINDFULLY

Rather than becoming lost in external experiences, like watching television, scrolling on your phone or working while you are eating, turn all of your attention to the food, savouring the flavours. When you see people eating mindlessly, while their attention is focused elsewhere, you may notice how quickly they eat without feeling satisfied afterwards. In fact, you may have had this experience yourself.

- **Sit down and enjoy your food:** Standing up to eat usually means that you are in a hurry. If you sit down, you will enjoy your food more – studies suggest that standing up or eating when busy and on the go can dampen the flavours.

- **Take smaller bites:** A small bite of food tastes just the same as a big forkful, but lasts longer. If you take smaller bites and chew for longer, eating will be more enjoyable!

- **Slow down:** It's true that eating more slowly makes you feel fuller. There is now plenty of evidence to show that it takes about 20 minutes for your brain to receive the message that you are full. If you slow down your eating, your body will notice that sense of fullness. Mindful eating will help you to connect and feel satisfied with that feeling.

- **Savour your food:** Experience joy when you prepare and eat your food – notice the texture, the colours and the smells as you cook. When you eat, savour your food, chewing it slowly and noticing all the flavours and textures in it.

Tip: Can you commit for one week to sitting down every time you eat something, whether it's a snack or a meal? This is a great step to help you connect and notice when you are eating and what you are eating. It also gives you a chance to pause.

Are you eating too much?

In menopause our bodies need less food – this is partly evolutionary. Scientists think that it's connected with the way we live in communities – as we stop reproducing, we have less

Mindful eating

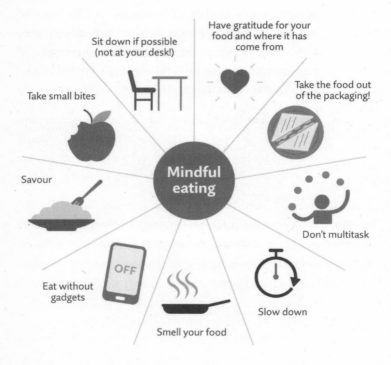

Sit down if possible (not at your desk!)

Have gratitude for your food and where it has come from

Take small bites

Take the food out of the packaging!

Savour

Mindful eating

Don't multitask

Eat without gadgets

OFF

Slow down

Smell your food

need for food. This also helps reduce competition for food, helping to support the survival of our species.

However, those messages between your stomach and your brain are a bit out of whack! If you have always eaten large amounts and loved your food over the years, your stomach will have got used it. It doesn't get smaller or bigger and stay that way; instead it's like elastic and can stretch and then come back to its normal size. If you are eating large amounts regularly, it gets used to being stretched and the 'STOP'! message from your stomach may be more a quiet whisper than a forceful command. If you can reduce the amounts you are eating over time, your stomach will start to feel that resistance sooner, sending a message to the brain that you are full. This is the principle that gastric band hypnosis works on – I don't particularly like this term, but I know that it's popular. I like to think of it as adjusting the settings in your stomach, so that it knows when it has sufficient food for you, sending a message to your brain to stop eating. Let's call this the full-o-meter for now.

Sometimes we need to relearn where to set it in order to feel satisfied. In this illustration I want you to draw the needle on where you think it should be for you. You call also print it off at www.penguin.co.uk/mindfulmenopause.

EXERCISE 74: RESETTING YOUR FULL-O-METER

- For this exercise you are going to access your Control Room (see page 53). Use your Calm Breath (see page 45) and your Hypnosis Cloud (see page 49), and your deepener too if you wish.

Full-o-meter

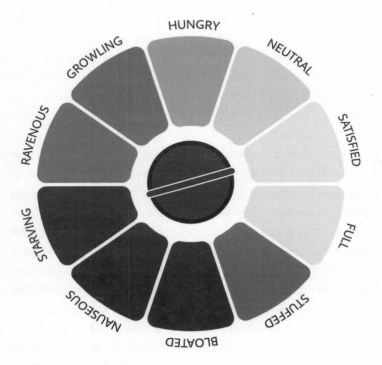

- When you are ready, bring the door of your Control Room into your mind, with the intention to turn down your full-o-meter.
- Then inwardly say your password.
- Once you have access to your room, your mind will follow your intention and take you to the full-o-meter.
- Notice the level it is set to and turn it down to where it needs to be for you to feel satisfied when you have eaten what your true self knows it needs to be well.
- Activate your willpower brain.

- Fix it in place.
- Remember, you can always return to this place whenever you wish.
- Open your eyes!

Now that your full-o-meter is set in that place, you will begin to notice that you are feeling fuller sooner, satisfied and energised with the changes you have made in how you choose to eat.

Moderation

This is not a time to give up what makes you happy! Healthy eating is important, but so is enjoying the things you love. Having chocolate cake every night of the week may be bit excessive – but you know that already. However, having a piece occasionally and eating it mindfully may be something to enjoy and relish. If you have a piece of cake it's not 'falling off the wagon'; it's stopping the wagon for a picnic on days that it matters to you.

Some of my clients come to me because they want me to 'stop them eating chocolate' or 'give up cake forever'. Are you really never going to eat a piece of chocolate again, or refuse a small piece of your birthday cake? The problem is that if a past habit was to eat big bars of chocolate, having one piece again will set off the old, conditioned response through association, unless you have worked on the realistic goal of moderation.

Tip: When you are enjoying something that you know you need to moderate, always make sure that you sit down, slow down and savour the flavour.

EXERCISE 75: ENJOYING WHAT MATTERS

Fill in the blank lines or add a few more!

Life is too short without . . .

_____

_____

_____

_____

_____

Tip: Try the ten-minute wait. If you want something just wait ten minutes, have a glass of water and then see how you feel after the ten minutes. If you still want it, go for it!

Movement

Movement is a fundamental part of well-being at any stage of your life, but even more so during menopause. How you choose to move and integrate movement into your life can change your experience in many ways. Your lifestyle may be changing, your motivation may have changed, your feelings towards your body may have changed, your body itself may have changed.

Everyone is at different levels of fitness, and I'm guessing that you already know what works for you and what doesn't, or what has worked for you and isn't now. Perhaps it's time for a radical change and to try something new? Is there a sport or activity that you have always wanted to try? If you are learning something new, it can also support your brain health. Keep going and create a long-term habit, make it your usual way of eating or exercising.

The important thing is that you get moving during peri-menopause! Looking after your body is part of your self-care. Regular movement can have a positive impact on your hormones, your brain health, your joints and your mood.

Finding the right exercise

Whether you are into team sports or are a solitary exerciser, find exercise that complements you in this stage of life. Did you know that tennis and cricket are the two sports that come out top in a study on bone health? Impact sports can be great for strengthening your bones and many sports clubs run sessions that get you started.

There is growing research to show that lots of intense high-impact exercise can work against you. If you are not used to it, you can put additional pressure on your adrenal glands, which may already be feeling the effects of lifestyle stress and the drop in progesterone. Instead think of exercise that can still have benefits such as yoga, Tai Chi, Pilates and brisk walking. If you have exercised a lot and are a big fan of aerobic exercise, this may be a big shift, but you don't need to get a sweat on to get your strength up.

It can be great to start in a group, as evidence shows that this helps with motivation and keeping something up for the long term. During perimenopause it's not uncommon to feel heightened social anxiety, which can be challenging if you want to join a sport that is a group activity. A simple way to build up your confidence is to use hypnosis.

EXERCISE 76: EXPANDING YOUR COMFORT ZONE

This exercise will help you expand your comfort zone in a way that feels right for you. The more you do it, the bigger your zone gets. Use the illustration as a guide. Sometimes it can be challenging to make that first step but when you do your circle gets bigger. Then you make the next step and it grows even more. When you continue like this your circle gets bigger and bigger, but you also gain confidence to try new things, creating an ever-expanding circle of confidence!

- Imagine a time in the past when you really felt confident. It might have been in a social setting where you felt very relaxed, or with a group of people who you feel confident being around. It can be somewhere from your past, or it can be somewhere in your present life. Just close your eyes for a moment, say the word 'confidence' in your mind and be open to what comes up.
- When that moment comes into your mind relive it, and experience that sense of confidence. Notice how it is. What you can hear, see, feel? Play it like a film in your mind.

- Squeeze your thumb and forefinger together and say a word that reminds you of this place and this feeling.
- Now in your mind go forward to a time in the future and imagine an event where you step out of your comfort zone. Say the word confidence, squeeze your thumb and forefinger together and experience in your mind how it feels when you are confident.
- The more you repeat this visualisation, the stronger the link between the word confidence and you feeling confident will be.

Tip: You can change the word from confidence to something of your own choosing. Think of a word that resonates with you.

Expanding your comfort zone

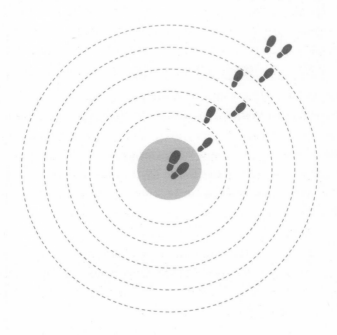

Patience

If you want to let go of weight, and you are embarking on your menopause well-being journey, be patient. If you are someone for whom weight has fallen off easily in the past, be prepared to be patient and persevere to get the same results. I believe that you will find the formula that makes you feel contented and fulfilled.

Usually my clients will do some research on:

- The best foods for menopause
- The most effective exercise

Then make a plan using:

- Goal-setting
- Hypnosis tools
- Mindful eating

Be patient with progress. You are on a journey to connect not just with your changing body, but changes in your life. By making a commitment to be open to change and opportunity, you are working towards your goal each and every day – it's okay to go to a party and metaphorically 'sit on the bench' for the day or go on holiday and sit on the beach for a week! This is all about optimising your well-being and bringing joy into your life.

'I am patient, kind and loving to my evolving body.'

Gratitude for your body

Your body has carried you from birth to this moment and experienced all the trials and tribulations, the joys and wonderment you have experienced. Your body may bear scars, love handles, stretchmarks, joints that have changed, a bum that is bigger, boobs that get bigger/smaller/droopier. Your body has adapted and grown since the day that you were born, perhaps it has seen you through illness, or childbirth, a wedding, maybe divorce or a marathon – it has supported your goals and achievements. It may have taken you travelling, it has woken up in the mornings, and gone to sleep at night, it has walked and walked, and hugged and loved. But it's not just the big moments, your existence, your body, is a remarkable feat of nature.

It also has an amazing system that diverts oxygenated blood to the brain when you are under pressure; it does everything it can to keep you alive and everything is finely tuned to keep you in the optimum health. It may have needed some support sometimes, but it got you here, to this moment and will continue to carry you. Without your awareness your body has given you periods, perhaps fed a baby, your heart has continued to beat, your lungs have continued to breathe, sometimes they may have had to fight for breath, but they rose to the challenge. If you put something in your mouth, you can experience taste, you automatically swallow. And music, it's pure magic – just think about what your ears can do not to mention a voice that can be a musical instrument. Your body gifts you an incredible range of experiences moment to moment, day by day. How often do you stop to notice it and offer it thanks?

'I am glad that you are my body –
thank you for all you do.'

How often do you stop to think about how incredibly glorious your body is, and what a marvel you are? However, you feel about your body, your mind and body are an inseparable team – if the relationship with your body has struggled in the past, now is the time to look at what an extraordinary job you have done together.

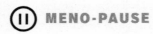 **MENO-PAUSE**

'I am glad that my body is supporting my journey through life.'

EXERCISE 77: GRATITUDE BODY MAP

I invite you to do this exercise, when you feel ready. It can help you to celebrate your remarkable and unique body. For this exercise you can take a photo of yourself either naked, in a swimming costume or bikini or clothed. Print it off on an A4 piece of paper – from both front and behind. Think about all the incredible things your body has done and continued to do. They may be big life events or they may be simple daily pleasures like your skin feeling the warmth of the sun.

Set some time aside to reflect and really start to see the miracle of your body, and the journey it has carried you on.

Then write those amazing things next to your different body parts. For example, these legs walk my dog, these breasts fed my baby, these arms give me joy when I hug people, my heart beats every moment of every day, this scar reminds me I am strong.

Letting go of weight and loving well-being is rooted in the magnificence of your body. Your body has cared for you, and all you have to do it care for it back. Whether that's supporting it with healthy eating, or simply loving it for what it does for you and for what it is.

Summary

Stop thinking weight loss and start thinking well-being. Use the tools in this chapter to create healthy habits and to meet the goals that you set. Be creative about these goals, not just in terms of size and weight but about how you feel about yourself, how you are eating and how you are living. Being healthy is more than weight. Celebrate your incredible body, each and every day. You get to choose to move and enjoy food in a way that supports your perimenopausal body and mind.

16

Putting It All into Practice

It's great to talk about female vulnerability and
mistakes, but you don't really see capable women
getting on with it. We don't sell the idea of being
an older woman to younger women. We don't
show that you are still the same brilliant, clever,
funny person – and now you've also got systems,
you can cope.

Caitlin Moran

Now that you have the tools, you can put them into action.
Use the list of exercises at the front of the book (see
page 10) and highlight the ones you found helped you the
most. You can bookmark pages if you are listening or add little
stickers on the pages that you want to come back to if you
have the book. You may have noted down some ideas in your
journal. I often find people come back and say, 'I use this all the
time,' or 'I love this' – it really comes down to what sparks in
you. You may find that one chapter speaks to you this year and
another chapter may speak to you more, maybe even a year
from now. What is important is that you know that all these
tools are a way to unlock what already exists within you. I'm
not creating something; you are awakening something.

How you put this into action is going to be completely personal and based on your life circumstances. You may be pressured for time around family commitments or you may have more time than ever. Think about all of this and know that there is no expectation, just the knowledge that small adjustments and changes can bring more balance and joy. There will be days that are simple, easy and happy – notice those and be glad for them. There will be days when it won't be so easy and I expect you notice them already, but now you have tools that give you permission to slow down, connect and let go.

Putting things into action can take time and there are five stages of change that you may find that you go through:

1. **Inaction.**
2. **Thinking about change:** This is making the decision to buy the book and read it. This is a commitment to learn something new about your experience.
3. **Preparation:** This is when you gather information. If you want to make long-lasting changes, preparation is really important. This is where you plan and do your research. Having knowledge to underpin your intention provides firm foundations and builds resilience. As well as reading this book, your preparation may be reading other books or researching aspects you want to know more about.
4. **Action:** This is when you start doing some of the exercises in the book and integrating them into your daily life – trying them out, seeing what works for you and what fits into your lifestyle.
5. **Keeping it going:** In time those changes will become habits. You can use reminders, sticky notes and your journal to keep you on track. Keep it simple to start with.

Checklist

Choose at least one thing from the list each day,
and see if you can cover them all in a week.

☐	Listen to a guided meditation	5 x Meno-pause today ☐
☐	Go for an Awe Walk	Listen to your affirmations ☐
☐	Tick something off your happiness prescription	Show some gratitude ☐
☐	Alternate Nostril Breathing	Add your own little slice of self-care

If you forget, come back to it. Keep returning to the exercises and tips that speak to you.

To help you, here is a checklist that you can download from www.penguin.co.uk/mindfulmenopause.

Do one every day from the checklist and add your own from your self-care circle (see page 172). If you have time, you can do more than one a day, but start off by setting yourself realistic goals. See if you can tick all of these off in a week at least once – with the exception of speaking kindly to yourself, which is something you can do every day!

Motivate yourself by setting goals, making use of micro-goals and visualisation tools – break down bigger goals down if you are feeling overwhelmed. Whether it's letting go of weight, feeling more rested, finding confidence at work or overcoming anxiety, taking small steps as well as big steps is a way of moving forward. However you choose to explore this time in your life, you are capable of so much, it can be a time rich with emotion and experience. The tough days will pass, but at the centre of it all you can connect with love and humour which is constant.

Finally, with everything you have learned, think of three words that spring to mind when you think of the word menopause now:

1. _____

2. _____

3. _____

Light your torch, connect with your heart, awaken your wisdom and step up to your power. You are the woman you have always been, and even more.

Resources

Here are some resources to get you started in exploring some more diverse approaches to menopause. There are further resources at:

www.mindfulmenopause.co.uk

You can download factsheets, templates, tracks and access e-courses that build on the information in this book.

Come and find me on social media:
Instagram: @mindful_menopause

Recommended Instagram accounts

@henpickednet
@janehardwickecollings
@larabriden
@libbystevenson.wellbeing
@megsmenopause
@menopause_doctor
@my_menopausal_vagina
@positivepauseuk
@saragottfriedmd
@the.hormone.doc

Recommended websites

gateway-women.com
henpicked.net
janehardwickecollings.com
menopausematters.co.uk
nationalmenopausefoundation.org
positivepause.co.uk
saragottfriedmd.com
themenopausedoctor.co.uk
u3a.org.uk

For more information on Kirtan Kriya, go to
alzheimersprevention.org/kirtan-kriya-yoga-exercise/
Use this video on YouTube to guide you.
youtube.com/watch?v=jfKEAiwrgeY

Recommended books

Hormone Repair Manual by Lara Briden
Daring Greatly by Brené Brown
Perimenopause Power by Maisie Hill
The Complete Guide to the Menopause by Dr Annice
    Mukherjee
The Hormone Cure by Sara Gottfried
The M Word by Dr Philippa Kaye
The Wisdom of Menopause by Christiane Northrup

References

Chapter 1
Elkins G.R., Fisher W.I., Johnson A.K., Carpenter J.S., Keith T.Z.
    (2013) 'Clinical Hypnosis in the Treatment of Postmenopausal

Hot Flashes: A Randomized Controlled Trial', *Menopause.*, 20:3, 291–298

Willemsen R., Vanderlinden J., (2008) 'Hypnotherapeutic Approaches for Alopecia', *International Journal of Clinical and Experimental Hypnosis,* 56:3

Saltis J., Tan, S.G.M., Cyna A.M. (2017) 'Hypnosis for Pain Relief', *Pain Medicine,* 571–574

Enjezab B., Farzinrad M.Z., Farzinrad B., 'Effect of Mindfulness-Based Cognitive Therapy on Menopausal Symptoms: A Randomised Controlled Trial', *Mazandaran Uni Medical Science,* 29:178, 85–97

Van Driel C.M., Stuursma A., Schroevers M.J., Mourits M.J. et al. (2019) 'Mindfulness, Cognitive Behavioural and Behaviour-based Therapy for Natural and Treatment-induced Menopausal Symptoms: A Systematic Review and Meta-analysis', *British Journal of Obstetrics and Gynaecology,* 126:3, 220–339

Linden, J. (June 2012) 'Discussion of Symposium Enhancing Healing: The Contribution of Hypnosis to Women's Healthcare', *American Journal of Clinical Hypnosis,* 140–144

Chapter 2

Digdon N. (2011) 'Effects of Constructive Worry, Imagery Distraction and Gratitude Interventions on Sleep Quality: A Pilot Trial', *Applied Psychology: Health and Well-Being,* 3:2, 193–206

Wood A.M., Joseph S., Lloyd J., Atkins S. (2009) 'Gratitude Influences Sleep Through the Mechanism of Pre-sleep Cognitions', *Journal of Psychosomatic Research,* 2009, 66, 43–48

Fox G.R., Kaplan J., Damasio H., Damasio A. (2015) 'Neural Correlates of Gratitude', *Frontiers in Psychology* 6:1491

McCullough M., Kimeldorf M., Cohen A. (2008) 'An Adaptation for Altruism: The Social Causes, Social Effects and Social Evolution of Gratitude', *Current Directions in Psychological Science.* 17:4, 281–285

Yu H., Gao X., Zhou Y., Zhou X. (2018) 'Decomposing Gratitude: Representation and Integration of Cognitive Antecedents of Gratitude on the Brain', *Journal of Neuroscience*, 38:21, 4886–4898

Zahn R., Moll J., Paiva M., Garrido G. et al. (2009) 'The Neural Basis of Human Social Values: Evidence from Functional MRI', *Cerebral Cortex*, 19:2, 276–283

Layous K., Nelson S.K., Kurtz J.L., Lyubomirsky, S. (2017) 'What Triggers Prosocial Effect? A Positive Feedback Loop Between Positive Activities, Kindness and Well-being', *The Journal of Positive Psychology*, 12:4, 385–398

Hamel M., Lajoie Y. (2005) 'Mental Imagery. Effects on Static Balance and Attentional Demands of the Elderly', *Aging Clinical and Experimental Research*, 17:3, 223–228

Renner F., Murphy F.C., Ji J.L., Manly T. (2019) 'Mental Imagery as a "Motivational Amplifier" to Promote Activities', *Behaviour Research and Therapy*, 114, 51–59

Chapter 3

Brent L., Ranks D., Balcomb K., Cant M. et al, (2015) 'Ecological Knowledge, Leadership and the Evolution of Menopause in Killer Whales', *Current Biology*, 25:6, 746–750

Davis S.R., Bell R.J., Robinson P.J., Handelsman D. et al, (2019) 'Testosterone and Estrone Increase From the Age of 70 Years: Findings From the Sex Hormones in Older Women Study', *The Journal of Clinical Endocrinology and Metabolism*, 104:12, 6291–6300,

Chapter 4

Tabibnia G., Radecki, D. (2018) 'Resilience Training That Can Change the Brain', *Consulting Psychology Journal: Practice and Research*, 70:1, 59–88

Snowdon D.A. (2003) 'Healthy Aging and Dementia: Findings from the Nun Study', *Annals of Internal Medicine*, 2:139(5 Pt 2), 450–4

Iacono D., Markesbery W.R., Gross M., et al. (2009) 'The Nun Study: Clinically Silent AD, Neuronal Hypertrophy, and Linguistic Skills in Early Life.', *Neurology*, 73:9, 665–673.

Benedicto E. (2015) 'Kirtan Kriya Meditation on Stress and Alzheimer's Disease', *Journal of Alzheimer's Disease*, 15:48, 1–12

Chapter 5

Sood R., Kuhle C.L., Kapoor E, Thielen J.M. et al, (2019) 'Association of Mindfulness and Stress with Menopausal Symptoms in Midlife Women', *Climacteric*, 22:4, 377–382

Woods N., Mitchell E., Smith-DiJulio K. (2009) 'Cortisol Levels During the Menopausal Transition and Early Postmenopause: Observations from the Seattle Midwife Women's Study', *Menopause*, 16:4, 708–18

Chapter 6

Bennett T. and Gaines J., (2010) 'Believing What You Hear: The Impact of Aging Stereotypes Upon the Old', *Educational Gerontology*, 36:5, 435–445

Critcher C.R., Dunning D. (2015) 'Self-Affirmation Provide a Broader Perspective on Self-Threat', *Personality and Social Psychology Bulletin*, 41:1, 3–18

Schmeichel, B.J., Vohs K. (2009) 'Self-affirmation and Self-control: Affirming Core Values Counteracts Ego Depletion.', *Journal of Personality and Social Psychology,* 96:4, 770–782

Cohen G.L., Sherman D.K. (2014) 'The Psychology of Change: Self-Affirmation and Social Psychological Intervention', *Annual Review of Psychology,* 65:1, 333–371

Chapter 7

Jalambadani Z., 'The Effectiveness of Mindfulness-Based Art Therapy (MBAT) on Healthy Lifestyle in Iranian Menopausal Women', *Journal of Lifestyle Medicine*, 10:1, 44–48

Barth C., Villringer A., Sacher J. (2015) 'Sex hormones affect neurotransmitters and shape the adult female brain during hormonal transition periods', *Frontiers in Neuroscience*, 9:37

Chapter 8

Light K.C., Grewen K.M., Ahmico J.A. (2005) 'More Frequent Partner Hugs and Higher Oxytocin Levels are Linked to Lower Blood Pressure and Heart Rate in Premenopausal Women', *Biological Psychology*, 69:1, 5–21

Chapter 9

Soosalu G., Henwood S., Deo A., 'Head, Heart and Gut in Decision Making: Development of a Multiple Brain Preference Questionnaire', *Sage Open Journals*

Chapter 10

Baker F.C., Lampio L., Saaresranta T., Polo-Kantola P. (2018) 'Sleep and Sleep Disorders in the Menopausal Transition.', *Sleep Medicine Clinics*, 13:3, 443–456

Otte, J.L., Carpenter, J.S., Roberts L., Elkins G., (2020) 'Self-Hypnosis for Sleep Disturbances in Menopausal Women', *Journal of Women's Health*, 29:3, 461–463

Gangwisch J.E., Hale L., St-Onge M., Choi L. et al (2020) 'High Glycemic Index and Glycemic Load Diets as Risk Factors for Insomnia: Analyses from the Women's Health Initiative', *The American Journal of Clinical Nutrition*, 111:2, 429–439

De Zambotti M., Trinder J., Colrain I., Baker F. (2016) 'Menstrual Cycle-Related Variation in Autonomic Nervous Functioning in Women in the Early Menopause Transition With and Without Insomnia Disorder', *Psychoneuroendocrinology,* 75:1, 44–51

Jansson-Fröjmark M., Evander J., Alfonsson S. (2019) 'Are Sleep Hygiene Practices Related to the Incident, Persistence and Remission of Insomnia? Findings from a Prospective Community Study', *Journal of Behavioural Medicine,* 42, 128–138

Chapter 11

Sliwinski J.R., Elkins G.R. (2017) 'Hypnotherapy to Reduce Hot Flashes: Examination of Response Expectancies as a Mediator of Outcomes', *Journal of Evidence-Based Integrative Medicine,* 22:4, 652–659

Thurston R.C. and Joffe H. (2011) 'Vasomotor Symptoms and Menopause' *Obstetrics and Gynecology Clinics of North America,* 38:2, 489–501

Chapter 12

Brandi M., Van Puymbroeck M. (2019) 'Enhancing Problem-and Emotion-focused Coping in Menopausal Women Through Yoga', *International Journal of Yoga Therapy,* 29:1, 57–64.

Stephens R.L. (1992) 'Imagery: A Treatment for Nursing Student Anxiety', *Journal of Nursing Education,* 1:7, 314–320

Chapter 13

Johnson A.K., Johnson A.J., Barton D., Elkins G. (2016) 'Hypnotic Relaxation Therapy and Sexual Function in Postmenopausal

Women', *International Journal of Clinical and Experimental Hypnosis*, 64:2, 213–24

Fuchs K., Hoch Z., Paldi E., Abramovici J. (2008) 'Hypnodesensitization Therapy of Vaginismus: Part 1 "in vitro" method. Part 2 "in vivo" method', *International Journal of Clinical and Experimental Hypnosis*, Jan, 14–156

Huerta R., Mena A., Malacara J.M., Díaz de Léon J. (1995) 'Symptoms at the Menopausal and Perimenopausel years: Their Relationship with Insulin, Obesity and Attitudes Towards Sexuality', *Psychoneuroendocrinology*, 20:8, 851–864

Chapter 14

Zhang B., Ma S., Rachmin I. *et al.* (2020) 'Hyperactivation of Sympathetic Nerves Drives Depletion of Melanocyte Stem Cells', *Nature* 577, 676–681

Chapter 15

Lebon F., Collet C., Guillot A. (2010) 'Benefits of Motor Imagery Training on Muscle Strength', *Journal of Strength and Conditioning Research*, 24:6, 1680–1687

Schreiber D.R., Dautovich N.D. (2017) 'Depressive Symptoms and Weight in Midlife Women: The Role of Stress Eating and Menopause Status', *Menopause*, 24:10, 1190–1199

Martin K.A., Hall C.R. (2017) 'Using Mental Imagery to Enhance Intrinsic Motivation', *Human Kinetics Journal*, 17:1, 54–69

Dunneram Y., Greenwood D.C., Burley V.J., et al (2018) 'Dietary Intake and Age at Natural Menopause: Results from the UK Women's Cohort Study', *Journal of Epidemiology and Community Health*, 72, 733–740.

Hewagalamulage TK Leel TK, Clarke K Henry BA (2016) 'Stress, Cortisol, and Obesity: A Role for Cortisol Responsiveness in Identifying Individuals Prone to Obesity', *Domestic Animal Endocrinology*, 56, S112–S120

Lombardo M., Perrone M.A., Guseva E., Aulis G. et al, (2020) 'Losing Weight After Menopause With Minimal Aerobic Training and Mediterranean Diet', *Nutrients*, 12, 2471

Dalen J., Smith B., Shelly B.M., Sloan A. et al (2010) 'Mindful Eating and Living (MEAL): Weight, Eating Behaviour and Psychological Outcomes Associated with a Mindfulness-Based Intervention for People with Obesity', *Complementary Therapies in Medicine*, 18:6, 260–26

Permissions

Chapter 8: Kate Figes quote, courtesy of Guardian News & Media Ltd

Acknowledgements

Sometimes it feels unreal to think that I've written three books, but not one of them would be possible without Julia Kellaway who is always there to guide me when I need her. She led me to the wonderful Jane Graham Maw, who took me under her wing and for whom I am always thankful. Sam Jackson, my editor, is more than just an editor – I've learned so much and I think I'm getting there! Dawn Bates, you took me through the most stress-free edit ever . . . a huge thanks. Dr Claire Harris, you are extraordinarily kind, the drinks are on me. Michele Donnison who has managed to make illustrations from my incomprehensible doodles. Thank you to Julianne Boutaleb, Jenny Tschiesche and Jane Hardwicke-Collings for your time so generously given. To all those who shared their powerful stories, thank you, especially the Cakehole Crew. A big shout out to my brilliant mother, Jenny, whose own wisdom is woven through these pages. And, lastly, I could never say thank you enough to Gordon and our boys, Fin and Rory, who supplied me with cups of tea, turned down the volume and respected the closed door when I needed to focus.

Index

Also by Sophie Fletcher:

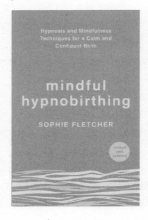 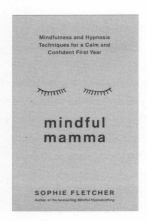

Mindful Hypnobirthing
Hypnosis and Mindfulness Techniques for a
Calm and Confident Birth

Using a powerful combination of mindfulness, hypnosis and relaxation techniques, experienced doula Sophie Fletcher will ensure you feel genuinely excited and completely prepared for birth. Reassuring, practical and based entirely on what works, *Mindful Hypnobirthing* is your essential guide to having a calm and confident birth experience.

Mindful Mamma
Mindfulness and Hypnosis Techniques for a
Calm and Confident First Year

Mindful Mamma is a reassuring and practical guide to help you to navigate the life-changing first year of motherhood. Using simple mindfulness and hypnosis techniques alongside MP3 tracks, *Mindful Mamma* is your essential toolkit to manage the physical, emotional and joyful chaos of motherhood.